THE POISON PATH GRIMOIRE

"Readers are taken on a captivating journey through the mysterious and often misunderstood world of poisonous plants. We are fully immersed in the forbidden gardens of herbalism, uncovering the secrets, history, folklore, recipes, and cautionary tales that bloom there. For those with a budding interest in herbal magick and medicine as well as seasoned green witches, this book is an indispensable resource that delves into the shadowy aspects of working with poisonous plants. *The Poison Path Grimoire* provides a fresh perspective on the ever-so-delicate dance between medicine and poison!"

NICOLETTE MIELE, AUTHOR OF *RUNES FOR THE GREEN WITCH*

"Coby Michael guides us into the forbidden corner of the witch's garden and reveals the link between our shadow selves and poisonous plants. Coby dispels fear about these plants and their relation to the occult without removing the magic and mystery, deepening our connection with these outcast plants. This book contains valuable insight into a lesser-known subject that will surprise and enlighten readers of all practices."

KATE FREULER, AUTHOR OF *MAGIC AT THE CROSSROADS*

"Coby Michael weaves a tapestry of myth, magic, alchemy, and spell-craft in this tour de force of plant magic. The recipes, rituals, and hands-on practices are clearly rooted in the author's own experiences, and they'll inspire you to deepen your love of poisonous plants and the wisdom they have to share. *The Poison Path Grimoire* elevates the practice of green magic to new heights."

NICHOLAS PEARSON, AUTHOR OF *CRYSTALS FOR PSYCHIC SELF-DEFENSE*

"Just like her aunt Circe in Homer, Medea was called by Apollonius of Rhodes a *polypharmakos*—'one who knows many drugs.' She was famously joined by Jason—a name given by Cheiron that also implies a knowledge of *pharmaka*—in the legendary search for the Golden Fleece. According to alchemical tradition, the Aureum Vellus was less a gilded ram's pelt than it was a priceless sheepskin parchment possessed of a potent recipe for a magical *pharmakon*. Coby Michael has proven to be a veritable *polypharmakos* himself, and *The Poison Path Grimoire* qualifies as nothing short of a genuine Aureum Vellus."

P. D. NEWMAN, AUTHOR OF *THEURGY*

"*The Poison Path Grimoire* is a mixture of science-backed herbalism, history, established poison path praxis, and deeply personal experience that is a well-constructed, desirable addition to any herbalist's library."

KAMDEN CORNELL, AUTHOR OF *THE TAMELESS PATH*

"Readers will be showered in the emerald gifts of poison plant sorcery and guided into connection with a host of plants, practices, and perspectives fueled by Coby's intense connection to this work and all it's capable of."

JOSH WILLIAMS, TRADITIONAL HERBALIST,
AUTHOR OF *SPIRITUAL HERBALISM*

"An excellent book for those wanting to dig their roots deeper into the gardens of shadow and wind their way down the crooked path with the help of its most famous and infamous green spirits."

ALBERT BJÖRN SHIELL, AUTHOR OF *ICELANDIC PLANT MAGIC*

"In his second book, Coby delves in-depth into the poison path, giving us many threads to explore from the tapestry of witchcraft and plant gnosis."

LAURIE BIANCIOTTO, AUTHOR OF *LA VOIE DU POISON*

"Examples of Coby's deep respect of and refreshing approach to verdant magic and lore are stunningly presented within the pages of *The Poison Path Grimoire*."

VEX BLÒÐSTJARNA, OCCULTIST AND
NORTHERN MYSTERIES SPECIALIST

"This grimoire holds universal wisdom related to baneful plants suitable to all type of magical practitioners and herbalists. Coby's philosophical approach to the poison path transforms this book into a guide not only for magick but also for contributing to spiritual development."

V. FAEMANA, ANIMIST HERBALIST, ARTIST, AND MUSICIAN

THE
POISON PATH GRIMOIRE

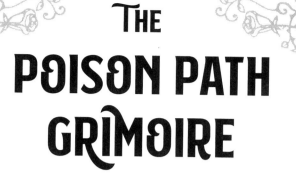

Dark Herbalism,
Poison Magic,
and Baneful Allies

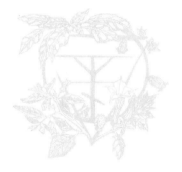

COBY MICHAEL

Destiny Books
Rochester, Vermont

Destiny Books
One Park Street
Rochester, Vermont 05767
www.DestinyBooks.com

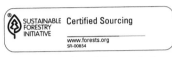

Text stock is SFI certified

Destiny Books is a division of Inner Traditions International

Cataloging-in-Publication Data for this title is available from the Library of
Congress

ISBN 978-1-64411-995-2 (print)
ISBN 978-1-64411-996-9 (ebook)

Printed and bound in the United States by Lake Book Manufacturing, LLC
The text stock is SFI certified. The Sustainable Forestry Initiative® program
promotes sustainable forest management.

10   9   8   7   6   5   4   3   2   1

Text design and layout by Virginia Scott Bowman
This book was typeset in Garamond Premier Pro, Gill Sans, and Legacy Sans with
Subversia and Nocturne Serif used as the display typeface.

To send correspondence to the author of this book, mail a first-class letter to the
author c/o Inner Traditions • Bear & Company, One Park Street, Rochester, VT
05767, and we will forward the communication, or contact the author directly at
www.thepoisonersapothecary.com.

Scan the QR code and save 25% at InnerTraditions.com.
Browse over 2,000 titles on spirituality, the occult, ancient
mysteries, new science, holistic health, and natural medicine.

✦

This book is dedicated to my mother, Kelley,
and to my sisters, Jenna, Jessica, and Melissa,
and to all of the other mothers, daughters, and sisters
who have been there for me along the way.

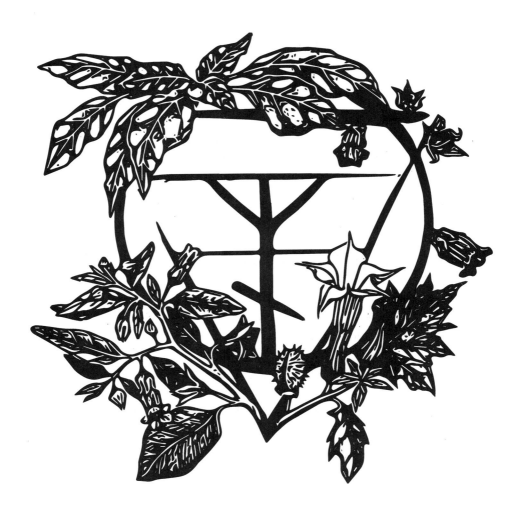

Artwork by Scarlet Loring

Contents

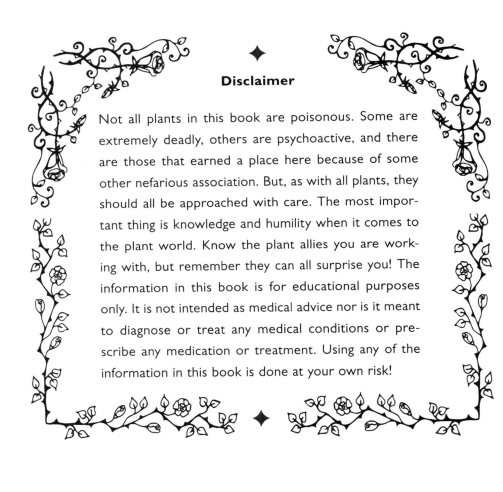

Disclaimer

Not all plants in this book are poisonous. Some are extremely deadly, others are psychoactive, and there are those that earned a place here because of some other nefarious association. But, as with all plants, they should all be approached with care. The most important thing is knowledge and humility when it comes to the plant world. Know the plant allies you are working with, but remember they can all surprise you! The information in this book is for educational purposes only. It is not intended as medical advice nor is it meant to diagnose or treat any medical conditions or prescribe any medication or treatment. Using any of the information in this book is done at your own risk!

Foreword

by Eimi OstaraMoon

I met Coby online through his classes and Instagram a few years ago, when I first started exploring the poison path. Though there were some great resources available at the time, such as *Veneficium* and *Thirteen Pathways of Occult Herbalism* by Daniel A. Schulke, or the Pharmako trilogy by Dale Pendell, and several longtime practitioners offered valuable advices through online blogs, I found Coby's offering of information to be most approachable. Whether it's the articles written for *Patheos*, his booklets on planet associations with baneful herbs, or his online courses on poison magic and flying ointments, Coby generously shares both technical and occult knowledge as well as his personal gnosis with poisonous plants and fungi. His passion to share the lost wisdom of obscure plants opens the door to a wonderful world of poisonous plants, fungi, and other forgotten or oft-overlooked plant allies for beginners and experienced witches alike. Attending his presentations, in person or online, is always like listening to a friend telling interesting yet informative stories.

Not only is Coby passionate about sharing the knowledge and magic of obscure plants, he is equally passionate about connecting all those who walk the poison path. Botanica Obscura, which Coby started in 2022, is a yearly online conference for lovers of plants and witchcraft who share a deep appreciation for dangerous yet healing flora, and sometimes fauna. It is a gathering of minds for those of us who walk the left-hand path, who are healers and hexers, as well as those who are simply curious. But more importantly, it is where friendships and connections are formed and more doors opened to explore other mysteries of plants and the occult. As someone who had just started on the poison path not long ago, I felt deeply honored when Coby invited me to present at the inaugural conference and subsequent events. That invitation allowed me to meet other amazing poisoners, witches, and plant people like Thomas Hatsis (a.k.a. the Psychedelic Historian), Harold Roth (author of *The Witching Herbs*), Josh Williams (author of *The Green Arte* and *Spiritual Herbalism*), Misha Nell (of Cypress Pillar Healing Arts in Sarasota, Florida), V. Faemana, Laurie Bianciotto, Matthew Venus (of Spiritus Arcanum in Peabody, Massachusetts), and too many others to name. I definitely thank Coby for opening that door to the poison path community for me.

And I am grateful for the friendship Coby offers. From the first time he asked for my opinion on one of his poison jewelry pieces through all the times he helped me navigate challenging circumstances, such as the passing of my father, Coby has stood by me as a mentor, colleague, and friend. He always held faith in me as I fumbled along the poison path, and he certainly inspired me to explore and expand my knowledge in the world of poisonous plants and occult herbalism.

If Coby's first book, *The Poison Path Herbal*, is the white rabbit that leads you down the rabbit hole of the poison path, then *The Poison Path Grimoire* is the Cheshire cat that explains the ins and outs of this mad and fascinating wonderland. Exploring the role of poisons and poisonous plants in various historical and cultural contexts, from vampiric herbalism to shadow work with baneful herbs, *ars aphrodisia*, and the use of poisons in traditional Chinese medicine, this book show us that we should not be afraid of poisons and poisonous plants, as they have been a part of our lives since ancient times. But with their deadly destructive and healing powers, they do demand our respect, and through this book, Coby guides us through the work of setting healthy boundaries for the sake of our physical and spiritual safety. *The Poison*

Path Grimoire is a continuation of *The Poison Path Herbal*, but it can also be read as a stand-alone volume. It is the perfect companion for anyone who wants to explore the esoteric side of the poison path.

EIMI OSTARAMOON, the witch and bee steward behind online shop Poison and Bee, LLC, started her journey on the poison path with a handful of *Datura innoxia* seeds and a dream of having her own Poison Garden on her farm in rural Texas. With the help of her honey bees, the garden has since grown to include baneful allies such as different datura varieties, henbane, deadly night-shade, and mandrake as well as various magical, medicinal, and culinary herbs. As a practitioner of alchemical herbalism, plant spirit medicine, and natural beekeeping, Eimi focuses her work with poisonous plants and honey bees by understanding their nature and needs and developing a harmonious symbiotic relationship between plants, insects, and humans. "Poison as medicine," both physically and spiritually, is the guiding principle that Eimi follows on the poison path. Eimi's website is poisonandbee.com and she can be found on Instagram @poisonplantwitchery.

Acknowledgments

It has been such a long journey since I began the work for my first book, *The Poison Path Herbal* (2021), and almost three years since its publication. There has been so much growth (and death) over these past few years, and I find myself in a place I never expected, but also exactly where I wanted to be for so long. It hasn't been easy, and the best and most visceral parts have happened in the shadows, away from the gaze of others.

I first and foremost want to acknowledge, honor, and thank the spirits that have informed this work and continue to guide me with whispered voices and inner knowing. I also acknowledge and honor the sacrifices, that which was given and that which was taken to make all of this possible. I honor and thank the ancestors for the blessings they have bestowed upon me and the ambition that has driven me to pursue this.

I would like to acknowledge and thank my sister Jess for everything we have been through and learned together. I had no idea what would be set in motion when we came back together, nor the incredible plant medicine practitioner you would become! Thank you for helping me become a better plant person myself, for reminding me why we are here, and for helping me get my wings back. While our journey has often led us to opposite corners of the world, you are always close to my heart, in the light of the moon and the warmth of the fire. I am so proud to be your brother!

The poison path community is one of the most unique, individualistic, genuine, and accepting communities of people around, with practitioners in all corners of the globe sharing an interest in working with powerful plants. It is a great honor to be a part of this network and to share it with so many intensely passionate individuals. The work we are all doing is something very special, and its full importance has yet to be realized by the wider magical community.

Thank you to everyone who has shared an interest in this work and supported me over the years. I am greatly humbled to be trusted with something like this, and I take it very seriously. Thank you to everyone who has read my articles or taken one of my classes, and a huge thank you to the support from the online community. It is with you all in mind that I constantly strive to push forward and elevate this practice through my own continuing education and experimentation as well as by sharing the work of others.

Poison path is just one name for a dauntingly vast umbrella of occult herbalism, and it is through the work of a multitude of herbalists, magical practitioners, and psychonauts that we are expanding our knowledge in this area, coming to a new understanding of our plant ally relationships, and reconnecting to the natural world. I would like to acknowledge, in particular, Harold Roth, author of *The Witching Herbs* (2017); Júlia Carreras Tort of *Occvlta*, author of *Land of the Goat: Witchcraft in the Pyrenees* (2023); and Thomas Hatsis, author of *The Witches' Ointment* (2015). These three individuals were some of my first influences when I began my own exploration.

Through this nebulous community of magical practitioners and plant people connected around the world, I have made some lasting friendships that stem from a deep level of understanding for and affinity for one another. I would like to extend my deepest gratitude to those who have supported me since the early days, who have come to be dear friends, and without whom I would not have had the support I needed when I needed it. Thank you to Nicholas Pearson, author of *Flower Essences from the Witch's Garden* (2022), for helping an orphaned author find a new and happy home! Thank you to Misha Nell of Cypress Pillar

Healing Arts in Sarasota, Florida, for your support in this world and the next, and for being a loving friend to all of the poisonous and venomous beings out there, including me! Thank you to Eimi OstaraMoon of the online shop Poison and Bee, LLC, for supporting me from the beginning as a friend and colleague; may our shared passion continue to grow in monstrous ways! Last, I would like to acknowledge herbalist Josh Williams, author of *Spiritual Herbalism* (2022) and *The Green Arte* (2022), for his work in animistic plant-based practice; you are truly the greenest human I know!

I would also like to take this opportunity to thank the publisher Inner Traditions/Bear & Co., for seeing the merit in this work and the need for more books like it! Thank you for taking a chance on this sometimes controversial topic that is near and dear to so many of our hearts.

BANEFULLY YOURS,
COBY MICHAEL
WALPURGISNACHT

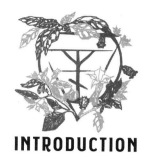

INTRODUCTION

Entering the Other Garden's Gate

Poison can mean so many things. In the words of the ancient Roman philosopher Lucretius, "What is food to one is bitter poison to another."

Powerful poisons known as toxins are found throughout the natural world. When a venomous creature releases toxins, it does so for defense and survival. For humans, poison can be many different things. It is found in medicine, magic, religion, legal discourse, folklore, and even mainstream popular culture. As a metaphor, it can represent everything from the spreading of an idea to complex human experiences from love to poetic inspiration. Humans are very much an active component in what poison is and what it is capable of.

The *poison path* is inherently individualistic. It is not a fixed way of working or a specific tradition of witchcraft, but the parallels between the two in both language and occult practice are undeniable. Throughout history, while the words change, these themes are spoken about almost synonymously and have been so for the better part of two thousand years. In this book, we will begin to explore in depth the intricate connections between the spirit of the witch and the essence of poison and how one can tap into these sources for occult exploration and personal empowerment.

The reader may notice that I have made a point to use lowercase letters for the term *poison path* throughout the book (when not being

1

used as part of the book's title). This contrasts with my use of the capitalized term *Poison Path* in my previous book, *The Poison Path Herbal*. Since the publication of that earlier book, I have come to feel that using capital letters implies that the poison path is its own tradition or that it is somehow distinguished from nonpoisonous pursuits. Whether or not to capitalize may seem like an arbitrary distinction, but the way we choose to speak and write about things says a lot more than we realize. I take a very eclectic and folkloric approach in my work with these plants, and thus *poison path* warrants no special capitalization. It's all just plant magic anyway.

I have been walking this poison path both personally and professionally for more than a decade. I myself found the poison path about halfway through my solitary magical journey, which began in my early adolescence. It is not my goal to create a magical tradition but to point out the multitude of intersections between the relevant concepts. It is at these crossroads, found throughout history and across cultures, that we can tap into a deeper universal wisdom. You don't have to be a witch or a plant medicine practitioner or even an herbalist to walk the poison path. Plants are fascinating in and of themselves, and they transmit gnosis outside of any context humans may try to place them in.

While much of the curiosity surrounding the plants found on the poison path is based on their medicinal applications and chemical constituents (see *The Poison Path Herbal* and recommended reading), my interest and expertise lie in their esoteric and spiritual qualities, their magical and ritual uses, and their consciousness-altering effects, which can help us to achieve plant spirit communion and personal gnosis. None of the information in this book should be taken as medical advice, and where specific medicinal information or action is included, it is done so only to provide a frame of reference for further personal exploration, should you so choose.

Which leads me to something I'd like to address right up front: *Dosis sola venenum facit*, "the dose makes the poison." Paracelsus, the father of modern toxicology, made many contributions to the study of medicine, chemistry, and more. However, on the poison path, he is best known for the preceding statement, which is a very important concept when it comes to approaching low-dose, potent, or potentially toxic plants and fungi. However, it seems to have caused some kind of fixation in the poison path community on "dosage" and "effect." Yet it is as much a philosophical adage as it is a suggestion of moderation when it comes to what we put in our bodies. My initial interest in poisonous plants came from seeing their poisonous nature reflecting their magical potential in an esoteric capacity. More physiological interactions came much later, and were not my initial interest after an adolescence full of uncomfortable psychedelic experiences. Through a *slow* and *gradual* exploration over the past two decades, I have come not only to understand new allies within the nightshade family but to establish a better relationship with my mushroom friends. As would be true for any other highly individual personal exploration, my best advice is to start at the very beginning and let the plants and your own body lead you on this journey.

My previous book goes more in depth into the chemical properties of specific plants as well as how to create formulas with them. It provides a number of recipes of my own devising as well as therapeutic formulations from the world's herbal pharmacopoeias. My intention there was to provide precedence for the use of plants like datura, henbane, and belladonna in modern medical practice as well as to provide thresholds for further personal exploration. You can find all of this information and more in *The Poison Path Herbal*, and much of the information in this book builds on that work.

As I did in *The Poison Path Herbal*, in this book I connect many abstract concepts and jump across cultures and time periods to express my version of poison path gnosis. The plant spirits transmit many things on many levels to many different people, and where I have brought in specific themes or existing mythologies, know that these are only containers for the deeper serpent wisdom that courses through this work. We can work with these plants to connect to a multitude of spirits and energies, and the faces I use to describe them are how they have manifested for me over the years. Yet the plants of the poison path are shapeshifters, and they are masters at reflecting us back to ourselves. To have a reflection, there must be both light and shadow . . .

Would poison exist without us? What is poison, and how have our ideas about it influenced our history? How does it continue to influence our daily lives? Why does this omnipresent and enigmatic substance hold such a sway over our attention? What constitutes a poison, and where is the line between poison and medicine? Poison has been used as a tool to control, to persecute, and to perpetuate a fear of the natural world. As an enemy of the social order, the crime of poisoning was anecdotally linked to women and called a cowardly act in public forums. However, men are no strangers to the use of poison. Poison as a metaphor is used to describe people and ideas that are a threat to the patriarchy and its henchmen, capitalism and religion. Understanding the philosophical side of poison, as a symbolic metaphor and occult force, is to begin at the original Promethean transmission at the Tree of Knowledge and follow the angelic corruption as it changes all it touches. Poison and witch are synonymous, both powerful catalysts of change, nondualistic in nature, a serpentine crack in the monolith of patriarchal oppression.

Late author, ethnobotanist, and poet Dale Pendell came up with the name *poison path* in his trilogy, which began in the 1990s with *Pharmako/Poeia: Plant Powers, Poisons & Herbcraft*. Pendell, an experienced psychonaut (explorer of psychedelic states of consciousness), was very familiar with mind-altering substances, Indigenous plant medicines, and drug use. He wielded the words *poison, venenum,* and *pharmakon* to express the nuances of distinction in this work, which investigates and explores the metaphysical and spiritual implications of working with various plant medicines that are also known for their "poisonous" qualities. The "poison path" was used to describe the alchemical extraction of entheogenic substances from potentially poisonous plants, specifically for their use in magic, ritual, and spiritual practice.

Pendell artistically presented the philosophies that make the framework of this path, as well as a system of categorization showing the wide spectrum of entheogenic experience. What a reader will quickly learn is that the poison path is more about this abstract and ambiguous concept of poison itself than a debate over whether or not a plant is poisonous in the absolute sense of the term.

Poison as an idea and concept comes with a lot of baggage, and working with mind-altering substances and the associated spiritual entities with this in mind is part of this exploration of occult toxicology.

The poison path is not only a place for the psychedelic or psychoactive plants and fungi that are well known for their mind-expanding abilities. It is also about those deadly, dangerous, and pernicious plants with the power to destroy. The poison path wouldn't be called such if the toxic qualities, both physical and spiritual, of these allies didn't hold some kind of special importance beyond their medicinal capabilities. Pendell does not miss this importance and spends three volumes exploring this idea in depth.

The poison path is rooted in occult pursuit, spiritual herbalism, and green gnosis. However, it is not an exclusively esoteric practice. The philosophies that one will find along the poison path will benefit all individuals, from the witch to the clinical herbalist. Poisonous plants can be just as magical in a clinical setting, and a holistic understanding of health and wellness is something that both the witch and the clinical herbalist have in common.

This book is written for the witch, the plant spirit practitioner, and the occult herbalist. If you have an interest in poison and its fascinating and dramatic history, this book will also be of interest to you. *The Poison Path Grimoire* is a collection of personal experiences, occult practices, and magical techniques to inspire and infect the reader with the intoxicating lightning strike that is poison path gnosis. While plants like deadly nightshade and hellebore are huge players in the poison path drama, the poison path is not exclusively a botanical practice, as you will see in these pages.

The Poison Path Grimoire is a magical tome, a book of "dark" herbalism, left-hand-path philosophy, shadow work, and spell craft for those answering the call to incorporate these power plants into their magical practice. The intention is not to present these plants or their spirits in a sinister or malicious way; humans have already done enough of that. In this work, I explore these contrasts because it is in the extremes that the most wisdom can be found.

The plants of the poison path are as much *bringers of light* as they are *children of the night*. All of the work here is meant to help heal, empower, and uplift. If you are like me, you will find as much healing in the darkness as you will in the light, and you will emerge capable of fully embodying both—because in the end, we are all rainbows anyway! We cannot honor the day by damning the night, nor hold night's blessing by cursing the light. I use the terms *dark* and *light* metaphorically to describe abstract concepts without any implied morality one way or the other. They are both just reflections in the same mirror; the face looking back is still ours whether the lights are on or off. These are my reflections, my shadows, and how they have manifested themselves in those around me through the work I have been doing.

It is my hope that you will come to better understand the spirits of the poison path, as well as deepen your relationship with your own plant spirit allies, by enriching your ritual practice through the insights and examples I have provided in this work. The following pages are all of the shadows I have collected over the years—a variety of occult practices and spiritual workings that can be adapted to suit any practice. I give you my poison book of shadows.

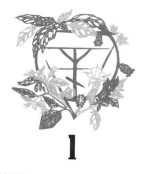

1

Lingua Serpentis

Speaking the Language of the Poison Path

*P*oison is an intrinsic part of the human experience, a concept that everyone has some understanding of. It is present in our oldest myths. The understanding of poison is chemical and substantial, and also metaphorical and allegorical. In the following section, I introduce some of the basic terminology relating to both the physical and esoteric understanding of this topic. Through working with these plants and fungi on both a physical and spiritual basis we can draw new connections that can aid us in our magical practice, personal healing and understanding of the natural world.

IMPORTANT TERMS

The following terms are commonly used by practitioners of the poison path, and knowing their meaning and context will help you in your research. Many of the resources of interest to the poison path practitioner are adjacent to the magical world, and further information comes from the study of ethnobotanists. Luckily, we are seeing more and more research and personal experience coming from practitioners also working with these plants in a physical and spiritual way. A more detailed look at these terms and others can be found in *The Poison Path Herbal*.

Alkaloid: One of the most important compounds occurring in plants. There are a wide variety of alkaloids occurring in a wide variety of plants (and not all plants contain alkaloids). Alkaloids are responsible for a plant's medicinal, psychoactive, and poisonous effects. They are secondary metabolites, or by-products of a plant's metabolic process. They can have a dramatic effect on human physiology. Caffeine, nicotine, morphine, and ephedrine are all plant-derived alkaloids, each one with a different effect. Alkaloids are generally categorized based on their effects or where they originate. For example, the tropane alkaloids are a group of alkaloids found in the nightshade family, which is of particular interest to those on the poison path. The most common tropane alkaloids are hyoscyamine, atropine, and scopolamine, and they occur in plants like belladonna, henbane, mandrake, and datura.

Entheogen: Deriving from Greek, meaning "to generate the divine within." Entheogens are plants and fungi that can create spiritual experiences through ritual application. There are many different types of entheogens, and they are all used differently and create different states of consciousness. Some are powerful psychoactives, and others are more subtle.

Ethnobotany/ethnopharmacology: The study of how people use the plants in their native land. In Indigenous and traditional cultures, health and wellness are viewed on multiple levels, with the spiritual and subtle aspects being just as important as the physical. *Ethnobotany* studies the way in which people have traditionally used these plants in medicine, magic, and religion in the plants' native or traditional range. *Ethnopharmacology* looks at the chemical constituents and medicinal actions of these plants and their compounds.

Ethnobotanicals

Ethnobotanical has become a catch-all term for herbs that are sold as "legal highs" and marketed for their relaxing, euphoric, and/or energizing effects. These plants, like kratom (*Mitragyna speciosa*), blue lotus (*Nymphaea caerulea*), and countless others, are legal in most places or occupy a gray area in regulation. In the United States, some of these plants are regulated by individual state governments. Just looking at Louisiana State Act No. 159, enacted in 2005, we see forty different plants with widely varying chemical composition collectively defined as "hallucinogenic" and declared illegal to cultivate, sell, or possess. The law was originally intended to rid the market of synthetic cannabis products like Spice and K2. It had to be amended in 2015 to allow for certain medicinal herbs that are commonly found in supplements and used in Chinese and Ayurvedic medicine but were inadvertently blanketed beneath this "war on drugs" policy.

Pharmacognosy: The study of medicinal drugs derived from natural sources. Pharmacognosy looks especially at alkaloids (see below), examining their medicinal effects and exploring how they can be made into medicines. We can apply some of this information to our own plant-based preparations. Where herbalism is more holistic, pharmacognosy looks at extracting specific constituents from plants.

Phytognosis: Plant knowledge, and more specifically the sudden realization of information that was not previously known and is believed to come directly from the plants. Plants communicate in different ways than humans do, and they send information to us in images, feelings, and sudden flashes of realization. Phytognosis comes only from spending time with plants and working with them on an intimate level.

Poison is medicine: Medicine can become poison, and to heal you must understand how to harm. This is profound wisdom, and important for all green practitioners to remember, whether they decide to work with the more poisonous plants or not. However, it is not strictly poison path wisdom. It is universal knowledge. All things in moderation. If that is all you take from your journey down the poison path, and you decide to turn back, that is totally okay. For those who wish to tempt the Fates and go deeper, there is more to be explored on the poison path than there is currently material written on it. We are just scratching the surface, and the witch occupies an important place at this revolutionary crossroads.

Veneficium: Poison magic. Closely related to *maleficium* (harmful witchcraft), sharing its connection to the arcane arts, and deriving from the Latin *venenum*, "poison." There is also a connection to the goddess Venus, as we can see in the root of the word. The line between intoxicating love potions and harmful poisons was often difficult to distinguish. Veneficium takes a particular interest in the occult properties of poison, using poisonous plants in spell work and magical practice and working with poison as an occult force. The term was popularized by Daniel A. Schulke in his book *Veneficium: Magic, Witchcraft and the Poison Path* (originally published in 2012), which continues to influence those who find the poison path through the practice of witchcraft.

PHILOSOPHIA TOXICUM

For me, the poison path has become an all-encompassing spiritual paradigm through which I operate, along with my spiritual allies, to express and manifest the current of witchcraft I am working with. While plants play a huge and almost exclusive role in this work, my interests lie not solely in the use of botanicals but also in exploring the very spiritual agencies within them. Through this exploration, my work has branched out in probably infinite different directions. There are so many different perspectives and places where poison lore, myths, legends, and superstitions pop up that we must consider them a global phenomenon. It is the larger role that poison and toxins have played in the evolution of humankind, both physically and nonphysically, that has become a major interest. In the following sections I begin to expand on some of these abstract concepts. I do this as a witch and an occult researcher, but also as an academic and plant medicine practitioner.

I have been writing and teaching about my experiences as a witch on the poison path since 2016. I have had the opportunity to get to know numerous other practitioners, each with their own way of working, their own perspective from which they approach this path. Few people choose to completely dedicate their occult pursuits to working with spiritual and physical poisons, for obvious reasons.

The poison path is animistic in nature, recognizing the spiritual forces alive inside plants and fungi. It is usually woven into an existing spiritual framework and used to supplement one's own unique practices. Poison path practitioners are all varieties of witches, alchemists, occultists, and plant-based spiritualists, and there is no right or wrong way to explore the poison path. In fact, calling it a *path* makes it sound like a closed tradition with clear boundaries. It is not. It is a *path* in that we choose to follow this pursuit wherever it may lead. It is not the only path for the verdant practitioner, and you cannot understand poisonous plants without first understanding their healing counterparts.

Although the poison path is focused on the occult nature of poisonous plants, it is a path of balance. There is as much emphasis on the antidote and panacea as there is on the toxin. This is why it is often also called the *crooked path*. One must travel the way of both the balm and the bane because staying on either side for too long has detrimental effects. To heal, we must go through our own ordeals, illnesses, and initiations and transmute our own spiritual poisons into power so that we can continue to heal ourselves and others. The poison garden also includes those baneful herbs that have an otherworldly, adversarial, or pernicious nature but aren't psychoactive or poisonous. The plants of the devil's garden and all forms of briar and bramble contain their own wisdom.

Practitioners of the poison path seek out plants that have been ostracized or forgotten by most people. The poison path is the way of the occultist and the witch, and while there are powerful physical forces at play, including a plant's toxic and visionary effects, the focus for the poison path is on the esoteric applications for these potent forces. In short, it is the study and application of poisonous, baneful, invasive, and demonized plants for their occult virtues and to connect with them as familiar spirits. This work helps one develop a deeper understanding of the *toxikon* or *pharmakon* and its transmutational power. It is a kind of plant alchemy, demonstrating that these master plant spirits work on many levels at once in a synergy that allows for their spiritual and magical effects.

> *Poison is a glyph for magical power itself.*
> DANIEL SCHULKE, *VENEFICIUM*

Much of the study of the poison path involves toxicology and its history. In the ancient world, the mechanism of poison was not understood on a chemical level. This did not stop people from using poisonous substances for medicine, murder, and magic. A large body of folk knowledge and legal discourse involving the idea of poison shows us this original understanding. Poison was a deadly and invisible force to ancient people. It could travel through the air, emanate from the evil eye, and contaminate anything nearby. The plants that were known to contain these malefic substances were thought to draw their poisonous nature directly from the underworld or the dead. Poison was seen as the great opposer—the antithesis of life force, but also sometimes its savior.

> *As Paracelsus noted, it [poison] is both omnipresent and absent in Nature.*
> DANIEL SCHULKE, *VENEFICIUM*

Poison is the original transgression, the intoxication of humankind through the apple of knowledge. It is the transmission of angelic knowledge to human beings to create something wholly different. Poison is that which is *other*, and that is exactly what the witch seeks to connect with. Contagion, miasma, and plague—accusations put toward many an accused witch—are all concepts related to the poison path. The church views witchcraft as a spiritual contagion, a toxin, infecting society with its maleficia. The poison path is an inherently rebellious path of self-discovery through trial, initiatory death, and shamanic visions.

The poison path witch is allied to the Promethean archetype, the light-bringer cast into darkness for stealing what was designated as only for the gods. We too can play this role, climbing into the branches of the world tree or descending into its roots to discover knowledge and to interact with nonhuman intelligences. The practitioner of the poison path achieves this through acts of opposition and entheogenic experience; both are a means of generating altered states of consciousness that result in spiritual experiences.

The Entheogenic Sacrament

These altered states are achieved through the use of entheogens, plants and fungi ritually prepared for their psychoactive effects. When honed through ritual action and clear purpose, these entheogenic states of consciousness confer deep trance states, otherworld travel, and communication with the spirit world.

Exploring the use of entheogens in spiritual practice is a large part of the poison path. This aspect lies along the path of *pharmakeía*, an ancient Greek term for knowledge of *pharmaka*, meaning potent plant-based preparations that were medicinal, intoxicating, and often potentially poisonous.

This is slightly different from the approach of the *venefica* or poison witch. The poison witch seeks to connect with the same forces previously mentioned. The focus here is more on the plant's baneful nature than its psychoactive properties, and accessing the plant's occult properties can be achieved without ingesting any plant material. This technique of traditional witchcraft is *atavistic*; in this way poison is used in ritual transgression or opposition to connect with numinous forces.

The Poisoned Chalice

The ultimate act of opposition, the poisoning of oneself* creates a powerful stir in the most primal parts of our mind. Allowing ourselves to come into contact with toxic substances goes against all our instincts of self-preservation. Even doing so symbolically creates a point of liminality that we can utilize when in trance to travel in spirit, communicate with other beings, cast powerful spells, and access knowledge through divination.

A symbolic act of poisoning oneself could be something as innocuous as floating the flower of deadly nightshade (*Atropa belladonna*) in a ritual chalice full of water or wine. While you are not in any actual danger, the act sends a powerful ripple into the spirit world. It says that this person is willing to approach death on its own terms.

The goal here is not actual death but ego death. Death of the self frees one from the constraints of one's present state of mind, situation, and personality so that deeper wells of consciousness can be accessed. This is the realm of the witches' Sabbath, the Wild Hunt, and the new perspective gained from hanging oneself on the world tree.

Other traditions also work with the energies of death, toxins, and contagion for their spiritual alchemy. The most common example may be the Aghori, devotees of the god Shiva Vishpan, the poison drinker. Their practices include ingesting toxic plants like *Aconitum ferox* and *Datura metel* with cannabis. Their way of working with the spirit world is similar to the thought behind the poison path, following the path of ecstasy and gnosis achieved through transgression. Related concepts of spiritual poison, evil air (miasma), and flying venom show up in other cultures as well.

Poison is a spiritual force as much as a physical compound, and here is where the occult wisdom in the poison path lies. It is at the intersec-

---

*I am by no means suggesting that anyone ingest anything poisonous. There are specific methods to this practice, and each is unique to the practitioner and the plant ally. This information comes through study, experience, and plant spirit communion.

tion of medicine and murder, somewhere in the realm between death and dreaming, and in the knowledge that poison is everywhere and nowhere. As a path of exploration, the poison path takes many different directions.

I don't presume to define anyone's path for them, nor am I under the impression that I have encountered everything the poison path has to teach me. All I can do is share what I see from where I stand and hope that others do the same. In short, the poison path is about connecting to the otherness that we all seek as magical practitioners. The plants that populate the poison path are an intermediary to that otherness, acting as its representative in this world. The path of the poisoner is to seek out these spirits for what they can teach us.

Poison is an alchemical force, and through its contemplation we become vessels for the venomous nectar, the forbidden fruit of knowledge. Through the art of in-toxication, we break the chains that hold us to our physical bodies and descend to Earth's mysterious depths, as well as deep within ourselves. It is in our own darkness that we find illumination. It is through transmuting our own personal poisons that we can claim sovereignty.

People often warn of the spiritual implications of working with poisonous and baneful plants. The concern is that the practitioner is somehow contaminated or tainted. They fear the darkness; they fear that if the sun sets, it will not return. Many of us found this practice as wounded healers, already carrying our own dark toxins. It is our affinity with these forces that calls us to this work.

ON DARK AND PRIMAL FORCES

The shadow is where most of our power lies.

Ivo Dominguez Jr.

When I talk about *dark* and *primal forces*, I don't mean anything "bad"; these terms simply point out important lessons and concepts that can be learned or discovered by those willing to look. While subjective perceptions of light and dark are purely human, it is important that we are able to understand and explore the nuances being presented to us. Exploring some of these perceived polarities helps us to better understand the full spectrum of the universe around us.

In a 2022 presentation, Ivo Dominguez Jr. noted: "Some things need to be embraced as they are. It is not our desire to make them harmless." That thought really resonated with me. Not everyone sees the shadow as a bad or unwanted thing. When we learn to live with our shadow, it can become our greatest ally. Some of us like being the monster in the woods, and this is not to suggest that we overly identify with this part of ourselves, but to say that we must really understand it for what it is. The shame and fear we are told to feel are the real shadows.

Darkness calls us to look deeper than what is on the surface. When we talk about "darkness," we are talking about things that are unknown, hidden, or other. Most popularly represented in shadow work, which seeks to understand and integrate these parts of the self, these "dark" aspects are parts of ourselves that we have separated from the whole because they are in contrast to part of the ego. For whatever the reason, whether trauma, conditioning, or a list of other possibilities, the conscious self must separate from these parts to maintain its version of reality. What happens when more parts of us become shadow than light? We can choose to stay in the familiar light of day and stay the same, or we can surrender to the shadow and embrace these parts of ourselves in new ways to foster transformation of the self. We are conditioned to call these parts of ourselves "demons," but they are in reality where our greatest lessons can be learned.

When we explore themes of darkness, work with entities considered questionable, or explore the depths of the underworld in spirit flight, we are simultaneously exploring our own shadow self. As Dominguez (2022) said, "When working with dark deities and spirits it is often the shadow self whose call is the loudest." The darkness always reflects what is within, and if we can get past the initial fear and discomfort of this confrontation, we can interact with this part of ourselves in a way that facilitates dialogue. The shadow is not something to be banished or neutralized; it is a depth of knowledge and transformation.

Witches celebrate their shadows. We honor the parts of ourselves that society and religion have told us to change and keep hidden. We revel in the transgressive power of our antinomian existence and seek to push the comfort zones of those who would try to constrain us. We can have a healthy relationship with our shadow self, which often manifests as the witch's familiar, with the same appetites and desires as its dayside counterpart. The shadow self, much like the fetch or astral double, is the ever-present nonphysical self, made up of your deepest dreams and oldest fears without the inhibitions of the conscious mind. The shadow self can be tricky and likes to confuse us as to its true nature. Working with "dark" deities and plant allies can help bring us into alignment with this work and offer additional support.

Embracing the darkness is not something that should be taken lightly, and it comes with its own set of concerns. Just like flying too close to the light of the sun, spending too much time in the dark can take its toll. The most important skill to learn when working with dark energies, spirits, and parts of the self is how to bring yourself back into the light in a way that is not traumatic. These are spirits of hard lessons, and when you approach the shadow, it takes you seriously. Think of it as willingly initiating your Saturn return and cramming all of its lessons into one moon cycle. Rebirth is a difficult process. We come into this world bloody, naked, and screaming, and that remains true for all of the little births and deaths we experience in our lifetime.

Working with plants, spirits, and themes that are perceived as "dark" attracts certain things to us. Confronting this reality elicits different responses in different people. It is important to remember that we not identify with those responses but act only as a dark mirror.

The left-hand path is about the elevation and empowerment of the self, and shadow work is essentially about self-empowerment. However, work on the self is not self-serving. Every community is made up of numerous diverse and individual selves, and to heal the self is to heal the whole. To uplift and to empower within is to uplift and empower without because when we learn to do this work for ourselves, we can help others through the process. Some of us are *light workers* and others are *shadow walkers*, and we need both to help the world heal. Like the dark goddess Kali, we can hold the darkness within ourselves and reflect the shadows inside others to help them heal.

Staying Balanced
while Undertaking Shadow Work

Shadow work can result in unseen energies manifesting in our lives. Without proper balancing, this can sometimes cause lethargy, depression, and intrusive thoughts.

To begin, we can look to the energetics of our physical space. Many of us who are attracted to this work are also attracted to the dark, sinister, and macabre, but it is important that we don't allow that energy to weigh us down, especially when we are going through transition periods and helping others in their healing processes.

Keeping live or cut flowers in the house is really helpful when it comes to lifting spirits and keeping the energy light. Regular cleansing, of course, is necessary; I prefer to use frankincense because I find it the most effective at raising the vibration of a space.

For me, one of the most important things lately has been my sleeping space. Every witch loves a spooky and sultry bedroom vibe, but sometimes all of the dark fabrics and dim lighting can attract some not-so-nice entities. A lot of stuff happens in the bedroom when we are asleep, and it is important to keep the energy in this room healthy. Depending on the time of year and the energy I am working with, I switch between black and white bedding. I also have lots of fairy lights strung around the room and hanging crystal light catchers. These factors have been really helpful in keeping a more uplifted energy in my bedroom.

Allowing natural light to enter the bedroom during the day is also really helpful because it moves stagnant energy. My bedroom window doesn't have the best light angle, so unless I open the window and let in the sun, the room can go days without seeing any light, which is not great for its energetic health. It is especially important during shadow work and intense periods of transition that we keep the energy moving within and around ourselves so we don't get stuck. Between the string lights and natural light, my bedroom is very rarely completely dark unless I am sleeping.

Because we sleep in our bedroom, this room is where much of our processing and healing occur. With the exception of personal altars to the self or ancestral altars, keeping altars outside the bedroom is helpful in setting and maintaining boundaries with the spirits you are working with and in promoting more restful sleep.

If you have a regular sleeping partner, it is helpful to have their permission for or involve them in the process of shadow work so that your energies are aligned. If you are seeing multiple partners in the bedroom for more than just sleeping, it is even more important that regular cleansing is practiced to maintain the health of the space. In speaking of partners, I would recommend limiting the number of new people that you bring into your space while you are doing this work because you can make yourself vulnerable and excite the shadows of the people you bring around you.

Shadow work can mean lots of different things, and there are many different reasons why one would want to work with the spirits of the underworld. Whether it is for shadow work or for spell craft, it is important that you approach all entities with respect and that you maintain the same personal boundaries you would if you were meeting a person for the first time in real life. Remember: You are the one who is in control, even when you choose to surrender.

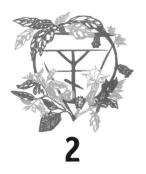

2

Poisons in Context

History, Mythology, and Occult Foundations

CHTHONIGENS: PLANTS OF FATE AND THE UNDERWORLD

The word *chthonic* derives from the Greek *kthon*, which relates to earth and soil. It refers to the subterranean world below, the crystalline matrix upon which reality grafts itself. This is the very fabric of the universe and the home of the Fates, a place of infinite potential.

The Fates were known as the Moirai by the Greeks, the Nornir by the Germanic people, and other names in other traditions. These enigmatic and primal forces are the personification of an inescapable law that binds us all: destiny. You may not believe in personal destiny. You may feel that it compromises our free will, but in a universe where even time and space are relative, it is hard to argue that there is *not* an unseen force guiding all of this.

As we know them, the Fates are a triad of women, sometimes beautiful and sometimes hideous. Regardless of their appearance or their names, they are powerful. We can think of the Fates as the guiding force of divine will, the enforcers of natural law. These figures are always female, and they represent various stages of life, death, and rebirth. Northern tradition holds that the Nornir live in the roots

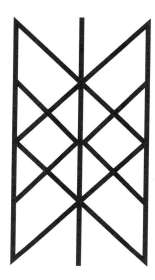

Web of Wyrd or Skuld's net, a symbol of the Nornir, from Jan Fries's *Helrunar: A Manual of Rune Magick* (1993)

of the world tree, Yggdrasil, where they carve runes into the wood to direct the course of events in the lives of the humans and the gods. In ancient Greek mythology, the Moirai are so powerful that even the gods heed their word.

Connecting with these primal forces in ritual is a serious task, and many practitioners say that it is a dangerous idea to call the Fates into our circle. I disagree. I believe that they are already there, and that when we practice magic of any kind we embody their work. The Fates spin, measure, and cut the threads of human existence. They are the weavers of the most important and powerful incantations. They are ones that hold the universe together.

Inviting the Fates into our circle, into our lives, is like holding on to a lightning rod in a thunderstorm. They can be the most powerful allies when it comes to co-creating our destiny, but they do so through "tower card" scenarios. Working with poisonous and psychoactive nightshades is a lot like this. It is important that we seek out the Fates only during the most important transition periods in our lives. After shamanic death, it is the Fates who sew us back together while they sing their songs. Once we are in sync with our Fate, there is no stopping us.

These feminine figures, shrouded in mystery, are perhaps the earliest archetype for the witch, and it is in their footsteps that all witches walk. Shakespeare modeled the witches in *Macbeth* after the three Fates. In their cauldron of potential, they brew mixtures of transgressive ingredients, influencing the lives of those around them.

All triple goddesses mirror the Fates in their triune forms. While humans are subject to their fates, the witch weaves her own, guided by these ancient spirits. The act of spinning, weaving, and working with thread calls forth imagery of grandmother spider building her web. Weaving has always been a sacred art, a vehicle for creation.

The three Fates could be seen as three aspects of the goddess Hekate. The queen of witches, Hekate was a Titan, more powerful than Zeus. The plants of Fate are the plants found in her poison garden, the Garden of Hekate or Circe. These are the plants that can bring intoxicating ecstasy or the silence of death. The one group of plants most associated with the Fates is the nightshade family (Solanaceae), whose members include tobacco, deadly nightshade, mandrake, and henbane, as well as many of our vegetables (not all nightshades are poisonous or intoxicating).

The Moirai of ancient Greece are three sisters, Clotho, Lachesis, and Atropos, and we see their names cast our classifications of the natural world. Atropos, the Inexorable, is the namesake of the genus *Atropa belladonna*, and her name was once used as a more general term for plants in this category, such as the formerly named *Atropa mandragora*. We see her name also in that of the alkaloid atropine, discovered in 1831. Atropos is the Fate responsible for cutting the thread of life, and she is called inexorable because no one can escape her. It makes sense that *Atropa belladonna*, or deadly nightshade, is named for her; if taken in too large a dose, it can cut the thread of life as well! The names of the Moirai appear in the animal world as well: Clotho, the Fate who spins the thread, is associated with the common hunter hawkmoth (*Theretra clotho*), and the genus of the venomous pit viper is named for Lachesis, the Fate who measures the length of the thread.

Nightshades have been connected to witchcraft, love magic, and murder for centuries. A deeper study of their associated mythology and folklore paints a picture of traditional European witchcraft. They can help us connect to spirits, journey in spirit, and heal on profound levels. These plants are historically considered dark and sinister, ruled by Saturn in traditional astrology. They are intimately connected to death, the underworld, the spirit world, and the occult. Working with them in ritual and ceremony as spiritual allies can help us delve into these areas, but we must work with them safely. There are many ways to do so, topically and sympathetically, in magic.

The plants in the nightshade family share themes of sex, death, and power. They are transgressive spirits, shadow workers, and death walkers that show us the hidden parts of ourselves and the world we live in. The spirits of plants in the nightshade family are earthly spirits, telluric and chthonic forces. We find their wisdom in the forest, the fertile earth, and the adversarial wilderness. They are not plants of the celestial realm. Untouched by the sky gods, they draw their power from the underworld. They are feral. They are feminine, and so is their magic—subtle, sneaky, and sometimes sinister, but not in a malicious sense. In astrology, *sinister* warns of an emerging influence, whether or not it is beneficial or detrimental. Nightshades are plants of darkness, not because they are evil, but because they are *other*. They have had to survive in the shadows and learn to thrive where others would fail. Does this sound familiar? It should.

Elementals, land spirits, and ancestors are all spirits connected to the physical power of a place. Genii loci, land dragons, and earth serpents are all examples of telluric or chthonic spirits. Some of them dwell on the earth and others dwell inside it. The jaguar, coyote, moth, and other nocturnal creatures also walk in this realm. They are the powers of night, darkness, and the unknown. As the luminary of the dark night sky, the moon also holds powers over the subtle and psychic realms. These forces are different from the verdant and generative powers at work during the day. These are the forces we encounter when we work with nightshades, the plants of Fate, and other baneful herbs. They are the forces of the underworld, the places untouched by the sun. This is the realm of the moon. *Witchcraft is the primal current of feminine rage, a lunar venom sublimated for centuries under the solar crucible of the patriarchy.*

Entheogens are plants and fungi that historically have had a ceremonial or religious importance. They are used in ritual to induce altered states of consciousness and help participants connect with the spirit world. As we noted in chapter 1, *entheogen* translates to "generate the divine within." It is plant spirit medicine, that which creates experiences of the divine. As a general term, *entheogen* is often used synonymously with the term *psychedelic*, though denoting a spiritual connotation as opposed to recreational use. We are starting to see, through experience and having nuanced discussions about these plants and fungi, that there are many different types of entheogens. Or at least different types of entheogenic use, as many of these botanicals can be used for various purposes. Thomas Hatsis expands on this idea in his 2018 book *Psychedelic Mystery Traditions*, in which he defines entheogenic subcategories like *pythiagen* (an entheogen used in a divinatory capacity) and *somnitheogen* (an entheogen that works via its sleep-inducing effects).

I like to use the term *cthonigenic* to distinguish work with plants related to spirits of the dead, familiar spirits, underworld journeying, and less celestially oriented practices. Like the other terms, *chthonigen* refers to how the plant is employed and in what context. When we are working with plants like henbane, datura, and even magic mushrooms, we are tapping into their chthonic qualities through entheogenic ritual practice. They are plants of the underworld that, when used entheogenically, create chthonic experiences. These might include working with "dark" deities, practicing necromancy, or working with occult forces for advancing one's witchcraft practice. Some poison path witches take the psychedelic approach, connecting with galactic consciousness and interdimensional entities, while others resonate more working with the consciousness of Earth and its spirits.

THE MAGIC OF POISON

The first transmission of venom took place in the Garden of Eden, a physical and spiritual corruption, according to the narrator of the tale. The intoxicating fire of heaven was given to us by the serpent, an ancient symbol of medicine, wisdom, and sexual liberation. Daniel Schulke writes, "This transmission of power originates with Samael, the transgressive Serpent-Angel and tempter offering poison unto First Woman. Indeed, the Hebrew name Samael may be translated 'poison of God' or 'venom of God'" (Schulke 2017). We are the venomous by-product of the world's creation, infecting and transforming all we touch. There exists an intimate relationship between the poisoner and the witch archetypes. Both poisoner and witch wield power, break taboo, and go against the norms. Many of the poisoner figures throughout history are women, legendary feminist folk heroes who were also believed to deal in the occult.

Poison magic comes from an interest in premodern ideas about toxins, both physical and spiritual, and from folklore and superstition related to contagion and protection against poison. Poison magic has been wielded to gain power and gnosis through inner transformation, plant spirit relationships, or more nefarious means. In everyday life, poison magic can be applied to transmute toxic energies, protect personal boundaries, and reclaim personal power.

While in its cruder forms poison has been used for harm, poison as a metaphysical concept has much more potential. *Venenum* means simultaneously "medicine, poison, and magic." Words for these things were often ambiguous in the ancient world, capable of multiple interpretations depending on the context. Applying this concept to poison magic, we can understand it as a means to:

✦ Work with poison as spiritual medicine
✦ Destroy harmful and unwanted influences
✦ Reclaim personal power

✦ Destroy harmful constructs, individually and collectively

✦ Enact cathartic or perspective-shifting experiences

✦ Work against the patriarchy, colonialism, capitalism, misogyny, homophobia, xenophobia, and so on

✦ Empower the individual

✦ Connect with occult and spiritual forces through taboo

Botanical, mineral, and animal toxins have played an important role in human history, with influence over politics, medicine, religion, and even our brain chemistry. Our earliest ancestors used poisons as a means of improving hunting by creating toxic projectiles or setting poisoned traps for more dangerous game. Poisons brought power and safety to those who knew how to use them, and this information was closely guarded in the ancient world. That secrecy created an air of mystery around them. People saw poison working but did not know how it worked or how it was prepared. The occult nature of poison, the secrecy involved in preparing it, and the pretenses under which it was deployed gave rise to many superstitions and apotropaic charms intended to protect against this unseen danger. It is this occult virtue and oftentimes inseparable connection to witchcraft that make poison a topic of interest to the magical practitioner. Poison has been used to kill, but also to protect, heal, enchant, intoxicate, and stir the passions. These are all things that magic has been used for as well.

One can travel many different avenues when considering the occult and magical implications of poison. Identifying spiritual toxins, transmuting unwanted or "contaminated" energy, transgression of taboos for gnosis, and practical magical applications are all within the poisoner's repertoire. Working with individual poisonous plants in the garden, studying their medicine, and connecting with them as magical allies teaches us that *poison* is a blanket term hiding many diverse effects. As a component in magic and ritual, poison brings power, and this power can be directed through associated symbols, spirits, and other occult correspondences. Here the line between poison and witchcraft blurs;

poison becomes an unseen and powerful force capable of healing and harming, as directed and colored by the intention of the practitioner.

In the following sections we will explore some of the historical, folkloric, and esoteric connections between poison and witchcraft.

A TOXIC HISTORY

Some of the earliest mentions of poisons can be found in Homer's *Odyssey*, in which the hero Odysseus poisons his arrows with hellebore. Hercules, the mythological hero, was believed to have invented the "poisoned arrow" when he dipped his own arrows in the venomous blood of the Hydra. Poisoned arrows and their effects are even described in the Bible. The tie between poison and arrows is so ancient that it is linguistically connected. The word *toxic* derives from the Greek *toxikón* and later Latin *toxicum*. The root of the word connects to *toxon*, the Greek word for bow, which is very close to *taxon*, Greek for the yew tree. Yew (*Taxus* spp.), in turn, was the preferred wood for making bows and arrows.

Veneficium (poison magic) and maleficium (witchcraft) were synonymous in the ancient world. Where there was poison, there was witchcraft. The Scythians of Asia Minor were feared throughout the ancient world. They were known for being fierce in battle and masters of sorcery and poison. They created a powerful toxin, called *scythicon*, and used psychological warfare to terrify their enemies. The Gaulish Celts were also feared by the Greeks and Romans. According to Pliny the Elder, the Celts poisoned their arrows using a formula called *limeum*, made with hellebore.

The ancient Thessalians were also feared for their poisons and practice of witchcraft. The witches of Thessaly, as they are known, are perhaps one of the earliest forms of the archetypal witch. One of the most famous is Chrysame, who is known for being responsible for the defeat of the Ionians at Erythrae, which she achieves based on her knowledge of poison, psychology, and ritual customs. An oracle had advised King Cnopus that he should make Chrysame the general of his army.

He listened to her advice, and Chrysame devised a nefarious plot to trick the enemy army into devouring meat that was full of hallucinogenic poison!

Throughout history, poison, like witchcraft, has been used to demonize, ostracize, and accuse individuals of heinous acts. It was just as easy to accuse someone of poisoning as it was to accuse them of witchcraft. The two are often found in the same trial documents. Not every poisoner was a folk hero. However, in many cases poison was capable of leveling the playing field, putting power in the hands of the powerless, and toppling regimes. Getting rid of an abusive husband, assassinating the next in line for the throne, usurpation, and the annihilation of rivals are a few of the causes poisoners have been enlisted for.

Poisoning was in vogue in Renaissance Europe. Alchemists, apothecaries, and herbalists would supply people with ingredients for poisons and other potions. Fortune-tellers and astrologists could be found in the same circles among people seeking to gain the upper hand at royal courts. Catherine de' Medici is a prime example, and she is often credited with bringing the "fashion" of poisoning to French court. The Affair of Poisons was a major spectacle in the court of King Louis XIV, in which a criminal underground consisting of a number of nobility led by Catherine Monvoisin was exposed. There were allegations of dealings in not only poisons but also black magic and love spells.

Many of the most infamous poisoners in history happen to be women. Interestingly, they all also seem have some kind of occult association or at least an accusation of witchcraft. We'll look at some of them later in this chapter.

FOLKLORE AND SUPERSTITION

A lot of the folklore and superstitions surrounding poison has to do with protection, detection, and neutralization of poison. Throughout history, poison was considered as much a spiritual corruption as a physical one. Ancient ideas about contagion, or the transmission of disease through "miasma" or evil air, influenced how people protected themselves. Death and disease were considered unseen evil forces up until a couple of hundred years ago, when we began to understand microbiology, and there remains an occult element to our understanding of these energies. Contamination, intoxication, transgression, and antinomianism—all of these concepts blend together in the idea of poison as an occult influence that can be accessed for magical purposes. By looking at how other people have thought of and interacted with this force, we can enrich our own understanding.

Countless charms, talismans, and other apotropaic devices have been created to guard against poisoning. Fossilized snake tongues, unicorn horns, and coveted toadstones were among the many magical charms believed to protect the bearer from any poisoning. While snake tongues are really shark teeth, unicorn horns are narwhal tusks, and toadstones are fossilized sea creature teeth, not all poison protection was purely magical. Mineral antidotes like emeralds, fossils, and mineral-rich clays were taken in the event of poisoning to absorb the toxins. Jade, agate, and amethyst were believed to counteract poisons in any liquid they were placed in. *Alexipharmaka* were formulas used to counteract poisons, while *theriac* was used as a remedy for venom. Theriac was an ancient preparation consisting of multiple ingredients originating as a cure for venomous snakes and mad dogs, later becoming a general term for an antidote to all known poisons in the same way the term *alexipharmic* described an antidote against poison or infection. Ambiguity between *pharmaka* and *venena* was common in the ancient world, and looking at the way these compounds are described gives us insight into our early understanding of poison before it became a catch-all term for anything deadly.

THE OCCULT

Poison is a primal force. It is everywhere and nowhere because everything has potential to be poisonous: plants, animals, minerals, excretions and extractions, spirits, energies. We even describe other humans, emotions, and situations as being "toxic" when they are harmful for us. Poison is anything that causes destruction to organisms that come into contact with it. It is contradictory, an antithetical by-product of creation. Poison is in opposition to life.

For any practice involving poison magic, spiritual hygiene uses the observance of taboos, cleansing and purification, and preventive practices to avoid coming into contact with forces considered tainted, corrupted, and infectious. Ritual bathing, avoiding certain foods, and working with sacred herbs were some of the ways one could prevent potentially toxic energies from building up in the body.

That is not to say that we should put all of our energy into protecting ourselves from poison. It is already all around us and within us. Our work is about developing a deeper and more personal understanding of these forces. That said, there are those few who focus on the occult aspects of this work. They seek out the taboo, whether it be poisonous plants, altered states, the dead, or darkness for personal power, spiritual gnosis, and connection to the divine. One prime example is the Aghoris, a sect of ascetic devotees of Shiva, the god of ecstasy, intoxication, and poison, among other things. These shamanic practitioners use trance techniques to connect with their deity, and they use psychoactive poisons, sleep in cemeteries, and use human remains in their rituals to initiate these states of consciousness through breaking a taboo. In witchcraft, this is called a "transgressive rite," meaning some widely held belief or common taboo is broken to create shifts in perspective and consciousness. There are less extreme ways of achieving this; when we work with poisonous plants, for example, we break taboo because for so long we have been told to stay away from them.

INFAMOUS POISONERS

In many ways, poison is synonymous with witchcraft. Each is an unseen force wielded in secret at risk of persecution and prosecution.

Poisons were once the medicines of the people—until the powers that be told us they were too dangerous for us to use ourselves, created synthetic analogs to sell to us, and took away our power plants. With poison magic, we reclaim our knowledge and protect those people and places that have been stewards of power plant medicine, keeping it alive. The industrial war machine of the patriarchy seeks to perpetuate the fear that we are safer avoiding the natural world in favor of manufactured security, but even today, just like always, there are people and plants that will stop at nothing to stand against that happening.

In the following section, we will go over some of the prominent and well-known historical figures and mythological and spiritual entities that are associated with poison. We can work with these figures, just like any spiritual ally, for a variety of magical purposes through their symbolic associations and our personal encounters with them. They can help us come to a deeper understanding of the energies we sometimes connect to when we work with certain poison plant allies or perform poison magic. They can be seen as potential patron spirits or at least supportive allies. That said, remember that spiritual entities represent different things to different people; a figure that seems like an ally to one may be an adversary to another.

Legendary Women

The female-poisoner archetype seems to float at the surface of the collective unconscious, and it makes sense, considering all the crimes against the feminine over the past few millennia and the ongoing struggle for equal human rights. Like Medea and Circe, powerful women who are both patrons of witchcraft and poisoners have been elevated to legendary status as folk heroes and allies. As we will see, many of them stood in direct opposition to patriarchy and the church. Some were scapegoated and all were vilified, seemingly just as much for being women as for being wielders of poison knowledge.

Locusta
TIME PERIOD: FIRST CENTURY CE

A Gaulish poisoner-for-hire, Locusta was commissioned by Agrippina, the former empress of Rome, to murder the emperor Claudius and pave the way for her son Nero to take the throne. Locusta succeeded in this, but she was scapegoated for the murder and imprisoned. However, she was freed by Emperor Nero and went on to successfully assassinate others, including Claudius's son Brittanicus.

Lucrezia Borgia
TIME PERIOD: FIFTEENTH CENTURY

The daughter of Cardinal Rodrigo de Borgia who would later become Pope Alexander VI, Lucrezia was born into the Borgia family, which dominated Renaissance Italy. Some call them the original Italian crime family, and indeed, a number of mysterious deaths revolved around the Borgias. Lucrezia was rumored to be a poisoner and is said to have worn a poison ring to parties. She fled to escape her accusers, but accusations of murder and sexual indecency allegedly followed her.

The Borgias and the Council of Ten (one of the governing bodies of the Republic of Venice) used a poison known as *la cantarella*. No recipes survive, but it may have included phosphorus, lead acetate, and arsenic or cantharidin.

Catherine de' Medici
TIME PERIOD: FIFTEENTH CENTURY

Catherine de' Medici, born into an Italian noble family, married King Henry II of France. As noted earlier, she is credited with introducing the fashion of poisoning to the French court. She is said to have had an obsession with poisons and potions; she employed alchemists and apothecaries and tested poisons on her subjects. She also had a notable interest in the occult and astrology and consulted famous diviners such as Cosimo Ruggeri and Nostradamus. She came under the suspicion of witchcraft when she had difficulty conceiving an heir in the early

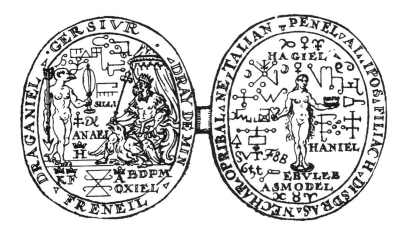

Talisman of Catherine de' Medici

years of her marriage to the king (she eventually gave birth to ten children). She is rumored to have practiced black magic and participated in satanic cults.

Giulia Tofana

TIME PERIOD: SEVENTEENTH CENTURY

In seventeenth-century Italy, divorce wasn't really an option, and many women suffered physical violence and other assaults on their personal agency from their husbands. Giulia Tofana, who admitted to at least six hundred murders using poison to help women escape from these situations, became an early feminist folk hero. She learned about poisons from an apothecary and taught the skills to her daughters, who went on to run successful cosmetics businesses, disguising their poison as a beauty product called Aqua Tofana.

Aqua Tofana

Aqua Tofana was originally formulated as a powder but was later replaced by a liquid. It was said that just four to six drops of the liquid could kill a man. When used correctly, it could accurately determine the timing of death, which would resemble that of a terminal illness.

The symptoms produced by Aqua Tofana were consistent with those of arsenic poisoning. Other ingredients included belladonna, antimony, lead, and cantharidin.

Mythological Figures

Poison as a literary tool represents forces that are primal, uncontrollable, and destructive. Its properties are magical and transformative. Poison plays a role in some of the world's creation myths and origin stories of the gods. Those figures with a connection to poison are set apart from others, whether wielding it as a weapon or a means of enacting magic. Through these stories we can begin to develop a sense of the connection between poison and medicine, divine and infernal, disease and healing.

The Hydra

The Hydra, a mythological serpentine monster, had venomous blood and many heads that would grow back when cut off. Hercules is said to have encountered this "monstrous viper-woman" and fathered three sons, who would become the ancestors of Scythia, with her. When Hercules finally kills the Hydra, he dips his arrows in her venom. In some depictions the goddess Athena is seen collecting the venom in a vial (Mayor 2003).

Medusa and the Gorgons

The Gorgons, whose name meant "terrible" or "fierce," were in some stories one entity and in others three sisters. They were depicted on ancient Greek vase paintings and sculptures as winged women with broad round heads, serpentine locks of hair, large staring eyes, wide mouths, lolling tongues, the tusks of swine, flared nostrils, and sometimes short, coarse beards. The most famous of them was Medusa, who is said to have once been a beautiful maiden, raped by the god

Poseidon and cursed for it by the goddess Athena. She is the patron spirit of those who have been broken and then punished for the damage done to them. The spirit of Medusa teaches us to revel in our monstrosity, to be terrible and beautiful. This rebellious spirit seeks to poison the patriarchy, and she has been called upon throughout history to bring freedom and power to the feminine individuals willing to wield her magic.

Gula

> *Gula, the woman, the mighty one, the prince of all women.*
> *His seed with a poison not curable,*
> *Without issue; in his body may she place*
> *All the days of his life.*
> *Blood and pus like water may he pour forth.*
>
> INSCRIPTION ON SUMERIAN TABLETS FROM 1400 BCE, ONE OF THE EARLIEST WRITTEN CONNECTIONS BETWEEN POISON AND WITCHCRAFT (FROM THOMPSON 1924, 26)

According to C. J. S. Thompson, writing in 1899, the earliest deity associated with poison is Gula, who was revered by the Sumerians as far back as 4500 BCE. Known as the "mistress of charms and spells" and "controller of noxious poisonous," she was also a patron and protector of medical schools at Borsippa and Sirpurra in ancient Babylon (Thompson 1924, 26). Gula was known as a great healer, but also one who could curse wrongdoers with poisonous herbs.

Samael

Samael is an archangel in Talmudic lore and is seen as an adversarial entity. A seductive and destroying angel who fulfills a divine function ultimately resulting in God's plan for humanity and their salvation. He is not evil, but tasked with the duty of acting as an adversary to humanity. He appears frequently in the story of the Garden of Eden in association with the Serpent that brought about the expulsion of Adam and Even. He is also considered to be the consort of Lilith and father of Cain. Samael's name translates as "Venom of God," and in this case the venom is knowledge or the act of transgression from angel to human. We could consider this extraterrestrial intelligence, the evolution of human consciousness due to non-human factors, the transference of angelic power in the story of the Fall, in which those angels who had been expelled from Heaven had children with the daughters of men, through whom the spiritual line of witchcraft was born, referred to as *witch fire*. Daniel Schulke writes, "The transmission of Poison first from angel unto tree, thence unto Eve and on from Eve unto Adam, conceals an initiatory formula of the Poison Path, the *transmigration of venom*, which accounts for the transfer and evolution of destructive principles from one body to another" (Schulke 2017, 147).

Apollo

A perfect example of the multifaceted nature of divinity, Apollo is simultaneously a deity of light and healing and a deliverer of plague and pestilence. It's common for spirits associated with medicine to contain both dark and light aspects, the capacity to heal as well as to harm, much like the dual aspects of remedies that serve as both medicine and poison.

Babalú Ayé (a.k.a. Omolu)

Babalú Ayé is one of the most feared and revered orishas of the Yoruba people and their descended traditions. He is a god of contagion and disease but also of health and healing—another manifestation of the common theme of duality in spirit healers. He is a divine plague doctor, tending the sick but also capable of causing illness to punish wrongdoers. In syncretic traditions, he is depicted as the Catholic saint Lazarus. Followers pray to Babalú Ayé for help in easing the transition into death when people are nearing the end.

Shiva-Vishapaharana

Shiva is the Hindu god of poison, intoxication, and ecstasy. The first term in the epithet *Vishapaharana* (the Lord Who Swallowed the World Poison) is *visha*, "poison." In the Hindu creation myth described in the *Rig Veda*, the holy cow churns up the water of the primordial ocean, releasing the poison *halahala*. It is so deadly that it is capable of killing the gods, so Shiva drinks it to save them. This is how he gets his blue throat or blue body—the color mirrors the blue color of aconite, one of Shiva's sacred plants. As noted earlier, Shiva's devotees, the Aghoris, consume *Aconitum ferox*, *Cannabis* spp., *Papaver somniferum*, and *Datura metel* for their entheogenic effects to connect with Shiva through trance (Rätsch 2005, 32).

St. Anthony

St. Anthony is the patron saint of all who are lost. St. Anthony's fire, a.k.a. holy fire, is another name for ergotism, the condition arising from long-term ergot poisoning and the burning sensation in the skin that it causes. The ergot fungi, which sometimes grew in premodern grain fields, caused mass hallucinations due to its alkaloid content. Ergot fungus is a naturally occurring source of lysergic acid or LSD.

Eitr

According to the Norse creation myth, as described in the *Vafthrúdnismál* of the ancient Poetic Edda, *eitr* is a generative venom responsible for all life. The frozen rivers known as the Elivagar are the source of this poison, which created the body of Ymir the first giant, from whose remains the world was made. While *eitr* is responsible for the creation of the world, it is also a deadly poison capable of killing the gods—another example of poison as a primordial creative and destructive power.

CHINESE MEDICINE AND *GU* MAGIC

I have found it helpful to look to cultures and traditions where the understanding of poison has evolved differently than it has in the West. Exploring the parallels and differences between concepts of poison, venom, toxins, and their occult counterparts gives us a better sense of this omnipresent force that has been with us since the very beginning. Poison as a concept evolved over many millennia, and our understanding of its mechanism of action is reflected in the language we use to discuss its nature. The following example looks to the East via traditional Chinese medicine, a system in which plants typically considered poisonous in the West are frequently used in medicine.

There are a few words with similar meanings to consider when discussing the concept of poison in Chinese medicine. *Du* is the standard Chinese word for poison today, but in the past it had a slightly different meaning: potency. Chinese medical philosophy recognizes the duality behind the power to heal and to harm, and when it comes to using potent ingredients like aconite to treat disease, it takes a different approach compared to Western herbal medicine, which tends to shy away from potentially toxic ingredients.

In the West, specifically in late medieval Europe, the separation between poison and medicine became more distinct in people's minds. This distinction crystallized in the early modern period with the rise of

Glyph for *gu* in oracle bone script, meaning poison and bewitchment

toxicology (Liu 2021, 6). In Chinese medicine, in comparison, medicines are reduced to single compounds with single actions. Rather, they were seen as "malleable substances whose effects varied considerably with the adjustment of dosage and processing" (Liu 2021, 56). The variety of drug preparation techniques, known collectively as *pao zhi*, can include boiling, steaming, stir-frying, soaking in brine, and more to reduce an herb's toxicity or enhance its efficacy. Dosage and method of administration are also key to causing medicines to work in a specific way.

As we see in the ancient Greek *pharmakis*, Amazonian *taitas*, African American *rootworkers*, and Anglo-Saxon *wortcunners*, in China individuals knowledgeable about medicinal herbs were also associated with the spirit world and the magical arts. Before modern medicine, the common person would have had some kind of general herb knowledge for survival, and that knowledge would have been passed on from generation to generation. However, certain highly potent plants were guarded with secrecy and known by only a few. The proper way to bring either the medicine or poison out of these plants at one's desire was a skill that put these wise ones in a position of power.

Chinese folklore and history tell of *fangshi*, healers who were sought for their healing preparations but also lived as social outcasts, echoing the paradigm of the venerated outsider. These individuals were tolerated both because they were needed and because they were feared. They combined alchemy, astrology, and the magical arts with their drug preparation practices, and their methods were seen as unorthodox. They occupied an inferior social position, but they also were summoned to royal court for their formulas. Like that of the *venefica*, or Western poisoner, their work delved into the occult and was shrouded in mystery.

Gu was seen as both a physical and spiritual contagion, a toxic substance with a malefic aura capable of killing from a distance, similar to the "evil air" or miasma associated with the dead in the West. While there were some wandering *gu* poisons in the form of demonic illnesses, as well as *gu* in the form of harmful creatures, the most feared form of *gu* was that manufactured by humans.

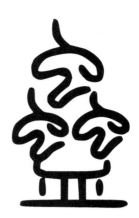

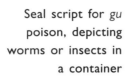

Seal script for *gu* poison, depicting worms or insects in a container

As it is in the West with poison, the concept of *gu* is associated with the feminine in the East. The *Classic of Changes*, a text on the Chinese divination system known as the I-Ching, displays *gu* as one of its sixty-four hexagram symbols. The pictogram represents essentially a destructive female power (supple force) bending and ruining what stands upright, namely male authority (Liu 2021, 70). *Gu*, like other feminine powers, was seen as hard to predict, difficult to capture, and capable of transformation.

Chinese history offers various examples of women being accused of practicing *gu* (poison) magic. Much like in the witch craze in the West, these accusations generally targeted women who were already social outcasts, exiled to the edges of the empire. Social class and regional family origin also came into play.

To create *gu* poison, the practitioner adds a number of venomous creatures to a container, but they also add their own malice to the mixture. In this way the poison takes shape via the destructive intent of its creator, becoming a kind of dark homunculi. People were believed to cultivate *gu* poison for personal power, to steal the wealth of others, to cause people to fall in love or lust, and to afflict enemies from a distance. In a scroll by first-century physician Chao Yuan Fang, we learn that "the affliction of others brings power to the owner of gu" (Liu 2021, 71). It was believed that outsiders, criminals, and other evildoers worshipped *gu* and its demonic essence for the power it brought to them.

Gu witchcraft is like a combination of psychic attack and the hoodoo trick of "putting live things" in someone. The drugs used to treat *gu* poisoning are many of the same used to expel demons. Potentially poisonous ingredients such as realgar, croton, aconite, and centipede are used to fight poison with poison via a violent purging process (Liu 2021, 72). In a "what doesn't kill you makes you stronger" approach, Chinese doctors believed "poison offered a powerful solution to target and destroy these obstinate but discreet pathological agents" (Liu 2021, 62).

Since *gu* is seen as a feminine or yin energy, it is remedied using fiery male or yang energy. Aconite is known for having fiery energetics and was considered a remedy for *gu*. A red snake that died on the fifth day of the fifth month, burned to ash, was another. This concept is also the basis for the Chinese five-poisons charm, a lucky protective talisman that depicts the five creatures with *gu:* a centipede, tiger/snake, spider, toad, and lizard. These are printed onto coins that are carried as talismans for protection.

3

Venefica

The Many Branches of the Poison Path

DEATH, DISEASE & CONTAGION: GRAVEYARD WORK

Our understanding of poison is connected to our understanding of death and disease. The dead have long been regarded as having nefarious and contagious spiritual qualities, with many taboos focused on containing and preventing those energies from escaping. Those spiritual manifestations of our earliest understanding of decomposition and contamination parallel what modern toxicology would describe microbiologically hundreds of years later.

Pestilent Spirits

In ancient times, the fear of *spiritus pestilens* (pestilent spirits) was not unfounded. In the time of Marcus Aurelius, for example, Roman soldiers conquered the city of Seleucia, then part of the Iranian Parthian empire. It's said that the Romans opened a golden casket in the Seleucian temple of Apollo, releasing a terrible spirit whose malicious infection soon spread far and wide. The Antonine Plague, as it's known today, was catastrophic, and perhaps the first factor in the eventual fall of the Roman Empire.

In later years, the Black Death led to three centuries of death, despair, and accusations of *pestis manufacta* (disease of diabolical origin)—that is, the intentional spreading of disease. In a study of the European witch-hunting craze, anthropologist Homayun Sidky points out the correlation between plague-spreader hysteria and the resulting witch hunts (Sidky 1997, 78). Both witchcraft and plague spreading were thought to be instigated by Satan.

Epidemics led to fanaticism such as self-flagellation, scapegoating, physical violence, and blame on the supernatural. Fears grew on the foundations of long-standing prejudices, leading to allegations that, for example, the plague was caused by Jews poisoning wells (Sidky 1997, 87) through the use of magical powders and salves. The paranoia spread as the death toll rose, and accusations infected all levels and branches of society. They were particularly damning toward anyone outside acceptable society, including not only women thought to be witches but also anyone proximate to death and disease, such as gravediggers, corpse handlers, lepers, and paupers. Many of these individuals were tortured until they confessed to spreading plague poisons and then burned alive.

Necromantic Plants

Fear of proximity to the dead extends to the plant world as well. Since ancient times, plants growing in a graveyard have been said to take on a baneful or "toxic" quality, receiving nourishment from the dead in the underworld. All plants and other material gathered from the graveyard maintain this baleful property.

Poisonous and hallucinogenic plants have long played a role in both funerary and necromantic rites. They were seen to have a connection to the dead not only because they were capable of causing death but also because their malefic qualities were believed to be a transferrable power originating in the underworld, creeping up into the plants. Herodotus described a renowned *necromanteon*, an oracle of the dead, at Ephyra, and scholars believe that various poisonous and hallucinogenic plants that grew in the area—deadly nightshade, black hellebore, and herbs said to have sprung from the sputum of Cerberus—were used in the necromantic rites performed there. Odysseus, the first mythological character to smear poison on his arrows, sailed to Ephyra to seek these deadly plants: "Ephyra in Epirus, near the River Styx and the mouth of the Acheron River of Hades, was a fitting place to gather poisons, since it was famed in antiquity as one of the 'gateways' into the realm of the dead" (Mayor 2003, 57).

Graveyard Work

There are many reasons to work with the dead and many methods for tapping into that connection. Let's begin with some simple guidelines for this sort of work:

- ✦ Set up protection (talisman, prayers, anointing oils, etc.) beforehand.
- ✦ Cleanse before and after (just like you would shower before visiting your living relatives).
- ✦ Draw a protective circle—a physical boundary to set the spiritual boundaries.
- ✦ Make an offering (incense, tobacco, honey, alcohol, cigarettes, candy, etc.).
- ✦ Set up a manifestation focal point or communication device (mirror, crystal sphere, candle, incense brazier) in its own separate circle.
- ✦ Be respectful and direct.
- ✦ Ask the dead for some detail only they would know.
- ✦ When closing (the most important part!), thank the spirits and say, "Good-bye, we're done now," before dismantling the circles and cleansing. To break the circle, simply draw a line through its boundary, breaking the spirit's circle first.
- ✦ Keep separate tools for working with the dead.

Plant Magic Necromancy

There are many ways in which plants can be associated with the dead, and in reality all plants are connected to the cycle of death and rebirth. The very soil that plants grow in is made of decomposing organic material that was once living.

One way to connect with death or the dead is through the help of plant spirits. They can assist us in many ways, including:

- ✦ To protect against/get rid of spirits
- ✦ To summon or banish spirits
- ✦ To prepare anointing oils, dyes, incense, and other tools for ritual use
- ✦ For spirit communication, divination, or perception
- ✦ For necromantic ritual
- ✦ To soothe the restless dead and help them move on
- ✦ For preservation or burial of the dead
- ✦ To heal grief
- ✦ To remember the dead and celebrate life
- ✦ To house spirits of the dead (trees)
- ✦ To open doorways to the spirit world

Thirteen Herbs for the Dead

In general, herbs and spices that are warming and/or sweet are pleasing to the dead. Cinnamon, chocolate, honey, allspice, and others (think fall flavors) remind us of life. In addition, the following herbs have a particularly strong affinity for graveyard work.

Apple: Symbol of the otherworld and of the Celtic "Isle of Apples" (Avalon). Symbol of forbidden knowledge (the Apple of Discord). A good food for the dead.

Chrysanthemum: A funerary flower, used for burial rituals and on altars for the dead. Symbol of rebirth, happiness, and vitality. Signifies that our connection to loved ones doesn't change upon death.

Dandelion: Used to summon spirits from the three realms and to help us connect with ancestors and familiar spirits. Can be taken as a tea or added to incense blends.

Elder: Known as the fairy tree (British Isles) or elder mother (Germanic). Said to be inhabited by spirits, witches, devils, etc. A gateway to the spirit world/fairy realm. Taboos about burning, cutting, and bringing elder wood inside. Dark and light aspects. An omen of death.

Gold copal: Important ritual use in Central and South America. Used in Día de los Muertos rituals to honor and please the dead. Pacifies spirits and protects the living without offending the dead.

Henbane: Strongly linked to the underworld. An ancient necromantic herb (one of the most important). Crowns of henbane placed on the dead. Psychoactive poison. Used for summoning spirits.

Life-everlasting: Used for contacting the spirit world, psychic healing, and ancestor work. Symbol of intuition and eternal life.

Monkshood: Known as the Angel of Death. Used by Aghori shamans in transgressive rituals to connect with the deity Shiva, a deity connected to ecstasy, intoxication, and poison. Through their use of poisonous and entheogenic plants and practices considered taboo such as their close work with the dead, these practitioners are able to enter trance states utilizing *Aconitum ferox*, *Datura metel*, and *Cannabis sativa* in their rituals. Common in monastery gardens. Hekate, as a patron deity of pharmakeia is associated with all poisonous and intoxicating plants. Monkshood has a close connection to this deity through its story of origin, appearing from the saliva of the dog Cerberus who guards the Underworld over which she presides in her role as Hekate Khthonia.

Mullein: Used for rustic candles/torches (hag's tapers or spirit lights) for the ritual circle. Assists in otherworld communication. Grows commonly in graveyards. (It's sometimes called "graveyard dirt," but it's really not unless it is collected from a graveyard, but in that case you might as well get the dirt!)

Rose: Used for divination and to increase psychic ability. Symbol of blood (red roses) and death (white roses). Symbol of secrecy (the thorny stems symbolize the hidden dark side to its beauty). Powerful heart medicine. Wood is protective against ghosts and other entities.

Star anise: Planted near graves and ancestral shrines and in temple gardens in Asia for protection and purity. Used to increase psychic power and "true dreaming."

Yarrow: Used to support psychic boundaries, intuitive ability, reception of psychic information, transmission of energy, and protection of energy field. Commonly grows in graveyards.

Yew: Long associated with death. Commonly planted in graveyards. Originally believed to absorb the miasma of the dead, to keep odors away, and to keep the dead from rising. Reputed to feed upon corpses, nourishing itself on death. The German rune for death, *eiwaz*, also denotes yew.

Cemetery Etiquette

A graveyard holds a lot of potential for sympathetic magic, transference magic, and more. Proper etiquette will ease the way. The following tips are by no means comprehensive or meant to represent the full scope of graveyard work; they are just some commonsense practices that have stuck with me and proven helpful.

- ✦ Place three coins at the gate or under the largest tree.
- ✦ Bring offerings that are biodegradable: water, tobacco, etc.
- ✦ Use plastic ziplock bags to discreetly collect graveyard dirt. They can be kept in your pockets and put on like a glove so you can do a quick grab and go if necessary. You could also use a smaller pocket-sized bottle as opposed to a large mason jar if you are concerned about drawing attention.
- ✦ Visit cemeteries during normal hours, and not during funeral services.
- ✦ If you don't know anyone buried in a cemetery, visit a couple times before taking anything and pay attention to how you feel.

If you notice a sense of heaviness, emotions such as sadness or anger that seem to come out of nowhere, or things suddenly going awry, this is an indication that the spirits of a place are not in alignment with your intentions and it is best to cleanse yourself and try again at another time or switch locations.

✦ Collect only natural objects.

✦ It's fine to take a small amount of dirt. Older cemeteries usually have worn areas where dirt is already exposed.

✦ Don't take any objects left by others at grave sites.

✦ Always pay for anything you collect. Leave coins, alcohol, or fragrant perfumes in its place.

✦ Don't look behind you until you have exited the gate.

✦ Cleanse afterward.

Material you collect from a graveyard is not bad or dangerous; it is simply a link to the dead. Keep it with reverence in a safe place. It can be one of the most versatile magical ingredients, used for protection, love magic, hexing, and help from the spirits with specific situations, depending on what you've collected.

VAMPIRIC HERBALISM: PLANTS THAT SUCK

The vampire is an ancient and powerful archetypal image, taking many forms over the centuries in countless myths of nocturnal and bloodthirsty creatures. The archetype of the vampire spirit can be found even in the plant world, where it shares an affinity with certain plants through symbolism, folklore, and energetics. Through the use of these plants, we can tap into the vampiric current, which can be applied to spell work, energy healing, and meditative ritual practice.

To understand the potential for working with the vampiric current in nature, we must understand the forces we are connecting with a little better.

Vampiric Qualities

✦ Drawing and absorbing life force

✦ Constricting, cold, paralyzing, asphyxiating

✦ Parasitic and epiphytic

✦ Capable of causing death

✦ Carnivorous

✦ Connection to the dead

✦ Connection to blood

✦ Mythological connection to the undead, nocturnal spirits, and vampire lore

How can we employ these qualities?

✦ Drawing out harmful energy, illness, and residual grossness (for example, using garlic cloves to absorb toxins and prevent illness)

✦ Diminishing disease spirits, diminishing a person's influence or power, or diminishing a situation or obstacle

✦ Draining energy from harmful and resistant spirits, starving them of ambient energy

✦ Protecting against nocturnal attack

✦ Glamour, seduction, personal power, influence, shape-shifting, self-defense

✦ Connecting with the powers of the night

✦ Personal empowerment

✦ Transgression and taboo, reclaiming power, and destroying patriarchy and its institutions

✦ Disempowering harmful witchcraft

Vampiric Energy Work

Most energetic healing modalities are based on recognition of a universal and infinite life force present within and around all of us. This energy goes by many names, including *chi, prana, od*, and *ruach*. Vampiric techniques work with this energy, but in opposite fashion. The energy is the same, but practitioners employ the opposite polarity, that which attracts and receives. It is the emptiness of space, the gap between electrons, antimatter—all the forces that consume and catalyze. Vampiric energy work may not resonate with everyone, but in the end, we are all working with the same universally abundant energy. The vampiric current, like other forms of energy work, is simply a way of connecting with and manipulating that numinous force.

Psychic Vampirism

The term *psychic vampire* gets used in a variety of ways that don't necessarily equate to the same thing. Sometimes psychic vampires are simply draining people with poor boundaries. This "type" is the most common, but it's not really a type because it's something we all might do during extremely difficult or dark events in our life, unconsciously draining the energy of those around us. At other times, psychic vampires are malicious manipulators, conscious of the harm they are causing. These reckless feeders practice nonconsensual energy draining and are usually solitary. There are also psychic vampires that are entities of an entirely spiritual nature, and they are the most dangerous.

Some people are born with this unique energy makeup, but we can also acquire it through occult means or through a traumatic disruption of the energy body. It often manifests as a pronounced deficiency in life force energy and a limited ability to produce enough energy on one's own to operate beyond a survival level. These individuals must find other ways to get the energy they need or they begin to experience a decline in health and overall wellness.

The unique ability to absorb and transmute energy into a force focused toward a specific goal or task can turn a deficiency into a source of power, and it is a form of energy work that can be learned. Working with one's own innate vampiric ability with the help of plant allies can be an effective technique for energy manipulation and spell work.

The Shamanic Vampire

The shamanic roots of the vampire spirit can be seen in key aspects of spirit flight and shape-shifting. Vampires are known for their ability to fly at night and to see with all the eyes of the creatures that make the night their domain. Sometimes a vampire will shapeshift into a wolf, bat, or other nocturnal creature or evanesce into a cloud of mist. In Romanian folklore, the vampiric creature known as the *varcolac* was believed to travel the spirit roads at night; it would fly up and drink the blood of the moon, causing lunar eclipses.

In Slavic countries, folklore tells of a witch-shaman called Dhampir who was responsible for discovering and battling vampires in spirit (Jackson 1994, 70). Indeed, unseen battles between the forces of good and evil are common in shamanic belief systems, and it is one of the responsibilities of the shaman to protect the community from pernicious outside forces. These same characteristics are seen in the medieval witch, and the nocturnal battles between benevolent and malevolent witches is a common folkloric theme in medieval Europe.

Modern practitioners will understand that the lines between good and evil are skewed, but there are harmful forces out there, and with vampiric energy, we can empower ourselves and fight fire with fire, like the vampiric shaman.

Court of the Night:
Connecting with Vampiric Herbs

Vampiric herbalism is one of the numerous lenses of plant-based spiritual practice. Not every plant radiates bright healing energy; some have a more shadowy nature when it comes to their interaction with humans. Vampiric herbs often slow things down; they draw energy in and conserve it; they are containing and constricting, often stopping the flow of life force energy. This power can either save or end a life, and it is what has made humankind fear and respect them.

These plants often have a connection through their folklore to vampires, as well as to witchcraft, devils, and creatures of the night. The further back we look in the history of these cross-cultural entities, the more we realize their shared origin. Which came first, the vampire or the witch? Or maybe the two are one, disguising itself as a shapeshifter the entire time? These herbs are linked to the stories of our allies in the shadows, and they can be a means of connecting with any number of vampiric spirits.

Many plants that are typically associated with vampires are used to protect against them, destroy them, or prevent them from rising in the first place. These botanicals contain deeper wisdom, protecting against spiritual contagion, miasma, energetic parasites, and toxic influences. Other plants in this category are predisposed to vampiric ritual and share characteristics embodied by the vampire. Still others are harmless or even medicinal, sharing only the vampiric affinity for the night and work done in darkness.

Plants that grow on a host plant, sometimes but not always drawing their nutrients from the host, are important allies for vampiric workings, specifically for their ability to draw in and store energy from the environment. One example is queen of the night/*reina de la noche* (*Epiphyllum oxypetalum*), a night-blooming epiphyte, which draws moisture and nutrients from the air around it. Energetically, epiphytes like this act as reservoirs, gathering and filtering ambient energy. Like quartz crystals, they can be distributed around the house for cleansing and protection, and they can also be charged with specific intentions. Carnivorous plants also have this quality of collecting and transmuting energy, which could be put toward a specific intention or general energetic cleanup.

According to tales from across cultures, a stake in the heart is a sure way to kill the undead and prevent them from rising again. The wood used to make these weapons itself has symbolic importance. Many types of wood are traditionally associated with vampire hunting as well as the fairy realm, including ash, hawthorn, rowan, and blackthorn. Ash is associated with the world tree, Yggdrasil, in Norse mythology, and rowan is an important magical tree often used for making rune staves and wands. Hawthorn and blackthorn are both believed to be gateways to the fairy realm. Blackthorn's sharp thorns are covered in a bacteria that can cause wounds to become extremely infected, adding to this hedge plant's sinister associations. Folklore also tells of rose wood being used for hunting vampires, and as we will see later, the rose is an important symbol for vampires today.

Brambles were often planted over graves in some parts of the world in hopes of containing the person buried there should they rise. Brambles, thorny trees, and other sharp plants are often associated with the crucifixion of Jesus of Nazareth, a kind of Christian plant correspondence that attempts to overwrite earlier folkloric associations with imagery of stigmata and other Christian symbols.

> After Rome became Christianized, the priests of the Church of Christ recognized the importance of utilizing the connection between plants and the old pagan worship that existed, bringing the floral world into active cooperation with the Christian Church by the institution of floral symbolism which should be associated not only with the names of the saints but also the festivals of the Church. (Folkard 1884, 31)

The Judas tree is said to be cursed by God since Judas hung himself from a specimen of this species. As punishment for his betrayal of Jesus, according to legend, Judas himself is cursed by God and turned into the first vampire—which is said to be the reason why vampires are averse to silver (in the *Gospel of Matthew*, Judas Iscariot was paid thirty pieces of silver to betray Jesus) and the sign of the cross. A similar fate befell Cain, brother of Abel, who is, according to the Old Testament, exiled, cursed with undying, and forced to wander the world marked as an outsider. Cain is often referred to as both the first farmer and the first vampire.

It is through the plants of the outsider/vampire that we step into our own power and out of the shadow of an unappeasable god. This is the power of transgression, a characteristic that one will find in all of the plants associated with witches, vampires, and the Devil. By connecting with these beings that we are taught to fear, and in many cases embodying them, we are able to get to a core of deeper truth within ourselves and our place in the cosmos. It is through these connections that we can align ourselves with transgressive forces to break taboos and reshape our inner and outer realities.

Many, many plants could be incorporated into vampiric workings. In the end, it is how we work with energy that makes it vampiric or otherwise. Certain plant allies support that endeavor and have an affinity for the energies we are working with. Whether it is the creation of servitors, charging energetic batteries, or draining energy for any number of reasons, these plants can facilitate and enhance those practices, teaching us new ways to work with the energy and opening us up to new types of spiritual experiences. Let's look at a few of them.

Blackberry Bramble
(*Rubus fruticosus*)

Blackberry bramble has had many taboos attached to it. It grows in dense tangled thickets creating boundaries that are difficult to move through without catching oneself on its sharp thorns. Brambles not only keep things out, but hold them in as seen in the grasping and tearing action of its thorns. Brambles were once planted atop graves to keep the dead from walking, creating a kind of natural cage. This grabbing, holding, and binding property belies this plant's vamiric ability to hold, absorb, and transfer energy. The brambles are made into wreaths and hung to protect against witches and other nocturnal spirits. Christian lore adds that the thorns represent the crown worn by Christ and the berries represent his blood.

A blackberry bramble arch was traditionally seen as an important liminal place, a gateway to the otherworld. People throughout Europe and North America passed their animals, children, and themselves under bramble arches for various reasons, from healing to asking the Devil for luck in cards (Watts 2007, 37). Offerings and a healing petition might be placed under an arch, and personal items of the sick could be hung on the brambles to diminish the illness by absorbing it through sympathetic magic. In a similar manner, the hair, clothing, or other personal ephemera of a target could be hung on the brambles to be diminished (worn away by the elements), sucking away the target's energy. This sort of transference magic, aimed at a target through object sympathy, is a very vampiric kind of magic. It can be used to transfer and diminish the power of disease, to hex and bind others, and to move and hold energy of all kinds.

As a vampiric ally, blackberries are helpful for those with anemia, a common problem for those with a low energy metabolism, because they contain iron and other minerals to nourish the blood. As a hedge plant, growing on boundaries, blackberry is associated with the liminal space between the worlds, a place the vampire knows well. Its brambles can be worked with to cast circles and strengthen boundaries when made into smoke bundles, and its leaves can be used in incense blends to open doorways to the spirit world or open roads to attract abundance. Like other vining tangling plants, it can also be used to create spirit vessels or energy traps; its intricate pieces can be placed inside a container to create a matrix for a specific energy or entity.

Because of all of the taboos associated with harvesting and eating blackberries, they are great for breaking taboos and going against the norm, as an herbal ally offering support to those who are working against the status quo. Eating blackberries in October, maybe even in the name of the Devil, in a simple rite to break a taboo and connect with transgressive powers and initiate change is a perfect way to tap into the spirit of this wild plant. Bramble teaches us to refuse to be cultivated and to grow how and where we please!

⚘

Blackthorn (*Prunus spinosa*)

Blackthorn is a sinister and sadistic plant for a number of reasons, so it is no wonder it is associated with the shadow. To begin, it is known for misleading people into thinking spring has come because it blooms at the first sign of warmth; its bloom is usually followed by what is called "blackthorn winter." It is often a harbinger of disaster to come, and an abundant harvest of its berries, called sloes, predicts an even harsher winter next year.

Like its relative hawthorn, blackthorn is a fairy tree and a hedge plant and has folkloric associations across the British Isles. In Suffolk and Somerset, it is said to be a death token, and it is considered bad luck to bring it into the home or to wear it (Watts 2007, 38). However, some people wear it specifically for protection, carrying it as a charm against all kinds of evil spirits, ill-wishers, danger, and misfortune.

In Ireland, blackthorn wood is buried with the dead, and the black-thorn staff or *shillelagh* is used by magicians and fairies alike. In the Balkans, vampire hunting stakes were made from blackthorn wood, which could be hardened by fire.

The thorns are covered in a pathogenic bacterium that can cause blood infections, adding to the already foreboding nature of this plant. The thorns were used for piercing poppets in harmful witchcraft. A folk cure for warts in England, and likely elsewhere, involved rubbing a living snail on the wart and then impaling it on a blackthorn tree for a nasty kind of transference magic.

As a vampiric ally, blackthorn can be a powerful partner, offering its wood for wands and other ritual tools, protective talismans, and spell components. More specifically, blackthorn wood is used to make staffs and wands known as blasting rods. These magical weapons are used for sending powerful hexes and also are extremely protective. The malefic use of these rods is an indication of their magical importance, not a limitation of their use. The berries or sloes can be used as the heart in poppets for hexing and other malefic workings, and the blackthorn tree makes a powerful familiar spirit and plant spirit ally when incorporated into solitary nocturnal rituals. The spirit of Blackthorn is considered to be bloodthirsty, and can be appeased with offering it a drop of blood before petitioning the spirit in magical workings.

Blackthorn is the door that leads to darker corners of the Otherworld and also within our own inner reality. It is a powerful ally for shadow work and shadow magic.

Rose (*Rosa* spp.)

The rose, whether red or white, is a classic symbol of the romantic vampire. It is seductive and beautiful but also capable of drawing blood. Like all flowering plants, it represents the impermanence of beauty and the idea that death makes beauty that much more precious. Its lush leaves and fragrant blossoms create a soft facade hiding twisted and sharp thorns. The rose is a symbol of inner and outer beauty. It is used in glamour and seduction magic, opening the hearts of all who behold it. Rose is a powerful plant all around, and one of the most effective herbs for attraction magic.

As a vampiric ally, rose is a power plant for all of these reasons and more. Rose is dynamic and draws all things to it through its beauty and charisma. It is both beautiful and dangerous, and it teaches us how to be both. The red rose represents blood, lust, and life. The white rose symbolizes death and the color of bone. Roses are sometimes planted at gravesites, where they can root down into the grave; when they bloom, that is said to be a sign that the person buried there is at peace.

St. John's Wort (*Hypericum perforatum*)

St. John's wort was once called *fuga daemonum*, "devil's flight," and it was known as early as the thirteenth century for its ability to cure melancholy and drive away demonic spirits. St. John's wort is a solar herb, and it is still used today to help balance mood and ease depression.

When working with plants and spirits associated with death and darkness, it is important to incorporate healing balms and solar herbs like St. John's wort into one's practice. Use St. John's wort to protect against vampiric attack and to neutralize dark energies. Its warm and uplifting nature can dispel some of the melancholy that sometimes arises from being a creature of the night.

Thorn Apple
(*Datura stramonium*)

Thorn apple is a species of night-blooming flower in the nightshade family. It is both vespertine and potentially poisonous. With its powerful tropane alkaloids, this plant has long been known for its medicinal and magical uses. It is said to have arrived in western Europe in the Middle Ages, brought by the Romany people, who used its seeds for divination and for their aphrodisiac effects. Thorn apple is associated with nocturnal flight and erotic dreams. Being both dangerous and seductive, it is a plant of the witch's garden and of the vampire.

Drawing Out Harmful Energy and Spirit Removal

The unique qualities of poisonous and baneful herbs can be employed for a variety of purposes, considering their Saturnian qualities and unique effects on the human life force. Saturnian herbs are constricting, cooling, and fortifying, and when we consider the poisonous qualities of certain Saturnian plants, which have a proficiency for drawing and containing energy, we can see the potential for use in various healing modalities incorporating the power of these special plant allies. Many plants of the poison path share the vampiric qualities of siphoning, transfer, and removal of harmful energies due to their Saturnian nature.

In this way these plants can be combined with energy work to target specific energies to diminish their influence and facilitate their removal.

In many shamanic and traditional healing modalities, illness and harmful energy are drawn out of the body and literally consumed and transported or transmuted by the healer. Oftentimes the illness or spirit is drawn out using the breath or the hands to direct and capture the energy. By incorporating the unique qualities of poisonous plants in topical application we can enhance the efficacy of these practices through the added power of the plant ally. Flying ointments and ritual oils make great tools for use in energetic healing, to either draw out unwanted energies or to contain and diminish the energies of an illness. Working on a subtle and energetic level, these preparations can be applied in specific areas, and also to the hands of the healer to direct and move things as necessary. These baneful preparations can also be employed to fight fire with fire and create an inhospitable environment for any low vibration, parasitic, or malevolent energies and influences.

Vampiric Formulas

When we think of plants, typically we think of life and growth, but a big part of that process is death, entropy, and decay. These powerful forces can be acted upon and incorporated into our magic. The formulas below were created to accentuate and utilize some of the unique vampiric properties we find in plants.

For these formulas, you can use plant material, essential oils, or a combination. For many of the ingredients, any part of the plant may be used unless specified. You might choose to make a base oil infusion with some of the ingredients and add the others afterward, and that is up to you. You won't find the amounts of ingredients specified because these are ritual formulas, and only a sympathetic amount is needed; if you only feel comfortable adding a small pinch of the baneful herbs, they will still do what they were meant to. I use sweet almond oil as the base for these formulas, but you can substitute other carrier oils as you desire.

Vampyre's Breath

Breath is life, and we breathe it into poppets and ritual fetishes to enliven and awaken them. The breath of life can be given, but it can also be taken away. This formula was created with that principle in mind. Use it to aid in the creation and sustainment of servitors and to impart vampiric qualities in objects.

- Fennel seeds or essential oil
- Dittany of Crete dried herb
- Mint dried herb or essential oil
- Mustard seeds and/or henbane seeds
- Wild lettuce dried herb
- Sweet almond oil

Combine all the ingredients.

Mark of Cain

Use this malefic hexing formula for siphoning energy and diminishing enemies, whether that's draining the energy of a harmful or annoying person or taking away the power of someone who is using it in a destructive way. The ingredients all have a dark, sadistic, and draining quality, whether through the act of asphyxiation or by their Saturnian nature. This formula is the black hole that draws all things in.

- Belladonna (dried plant material)
- Hellebore (dried plant material)
- Poison hemlock (dried plant material) ☠ deadly poison; use extra caution if handling fresh plant material ☠
- Sweet almond oil

Combine all the ingredients. I like to use belladonna infused oil combined with sweet almond oil as my base, mixing my 1:10 belladonna infusion 50:50 with sweet almond oil. Then I add the other ingredients, including dried belladonna herb, to the individual and mother bottles.

Blood of Seraphim

This formula has the color and consistency of human blood and also a sweet and tempting smell, making it a perfect sanguine offertory oleum for enlivening objects, feeding or attracting spirits, and reddening bones. It can be used in rituals in the place of blood with the same impact. Just the sight of blood is enough to trigger primal changes deep in our mind, and this formula gets that job done.

- Cacao powder
- Dragon's blood resin powder
- Red sandalwood powder
- Sweet almond oil
- Blood orange essential oil
- Dragon's blood fragrance oil
- Blood root powder or pieces

Infuse the cacao powder, dragon's blood resin powder, and red sandalwood powder in sweet almond oil for 1 to 2 weeks. Strain, then add blood orange and dragon's blood oils and a small amount of blood root.

Vampiric Drawing Salve Recipe

This recipe was inspired by black drawing salves, which are used medicinally for a variety of healing purposes. However, in this case the "drawing" is more related to the attractive and vampiric nature of this formulation. It can be used as an anointing oil for a variety of vampiric workings, from glamour magic to gathering and storing energy. Depending on how you work with it, this formula could effect either baneful or beneficial workings, from diminishing a man's nature to diminishing the power of an illness.

- **Poison hemlock ☠ deadly poison; use extra caution if handling fresh plant material ☠**
- **Rose petals**
- **Cinquefoil**
- **Oak moss**
- **Comfrey leaves**
- **Cacao powder**
- **Dragon's blood resin powder**
- **Activated charcoal**
- **Sweet almond oil**
- **Beeswax**

For the base of the salve, infuse the plant material and charcoal in the sweet almond oil. (Only small amounts of plant material are needed.) Then warm the oil with beeswax (about one third of the amount of oil you are preparing) until the two are well combined; let cool.*

The following incantation was adapted from John George Hohman's 1828 work *Pow-Wows or Long Lost Friend*. It was originally intended to "diminish a man of greater strength and vitality," and I find it has potential for a lot of other things too. It can be spoken when using the ointment as a vampiric formula for anointing people, ritual objects, or other forms of ritual application.

I *(your name)* breathe upon thee. Three drops of blood I take from thee: the first out of thy heart, the second out of thy liver, and the third out of thy vital powers; and in this I deprive thee of thy strength and thou art diminished. Hbbi massa danti Lantien. I.I.I.

---

*For more information on salve making including the witches' flying ointment see *The Poison Path Herbal* (2021).

ARS APHRODISIA: THE ARTS OF VENUS

Many of the original "poisons" were potions intended for love magic. Some employed another category of plant that has earned its place in the poison garden: the psychoactive aphrodisiac. Not all aphrodisiacs are psychoactive, and some are only mildly so. However, they all have the ability to poison the mind, enrapture the senses, and warp the perceptions of those under their influence. Depending on the circumstances, an aphrodisiac can quickly turn from balm to bane. Taking away another person's ability to give (or not give) consent is the first step down a malefic road, and this kind of behavior cannot be condoned.

Historically, aphrodisiac love potions, or *pocula amatoria*, were prevalent. Composed of intoxicating and "poisonous" ingredients like mandrake, opium poppy, belladonna, cannabis, and more, these were premodern versions of date-rape drugs and often became the subject of criminal litigation. For a time, it was the intention or status of the user that proved guilt or innocence. Usually, money, gender, and social standing were the determining factors on the acceptability of using these preparations. Being drugged by someone of a higher social standing was seen as harmless or as a favor. The psychoactive effects of hypnotic and deliriant plants from the nightshade family were seen as part of a love potion's magic, though they could easily lead to an overdose. Nonetheless, these preparations have survived from antiquity, thriving in the aristocracy, and some are still used as aphrodisiacs today.

As with all things, plants exist on a spectrum. On one extreme end are things like devil's breath, a hypnotic and deliriant compound made from the scopolamine extracted from plants like angel's trumpet (*Brugmansia* spp.). It is not plant medicine but isolated alkaloids used solely to hurt people (see page 109). It has a history of use by criminals to make their victims compliant.

But this is the sinister side of the aphrodisiac, and it has more to offer. Angel's trumpet and its close relatives in the *Datura* genus are known for their aphrodisiac effects, which derive at least in part from their scopolamine content. In small doses, among consenting individuals, these plants are sometimes used to lower inhibitions and experience altered sexual consciousness. In larger doses, they are hypnotic and deliriant, and also potentially deadly. Yet they have been used as ingredients in love potions around the world, including in the Americas, Europe, and India. One example is the formula known as *jugo de toloache*, which comes from Mexico and is also sold in botanicas in the United States. It is a manipulative love potion made with *Datura innoxia* and able to give one influence over another person they desire.

On the opposite end of the spectrum would be things like cacao (*Theobroma cacao*), rose (*Rosa* spp.), and cannabis (*Cannabis sativa*), which are recognized around the world for their aphrodisiac effects and association with love and intimacy. These plant allies carry little to no risk, and we can work with them entheogenically to open the heart and connect with Venusian energies.

While many aphrodisiacs are innocuous enough, and many can be taken regularly to support overall health, there are those that occupy a middle road. We find the nightshade family in this twilight realm of the witch and the poisoner. These baneful herbs, best known for the harm they are capable of causing, also have relaxing, intoxicating, and aphrodisiac effects. When combined with other aphrodisiac herbs, they can be powerful allies for ecstatic trance, rites of a sexual nature, and directing the powerful energies that arise when we are aroused. We can work with them for celebratory rituals, spells for specific intentions, or rituals for self-love and healing. When we begin to connect the plants to specific states of consciousness, the potential is endless for how we can enhance our magical practice by altering our consciousness, even just slightly.

Beneath their sinister facade, the nightshade family is full of aphrodisiac herbs. From ashwagandha to henbane, all the most infamous nightshades have also been used for their aphrodisiac effects. They offer intoxicating inebriation, so much so that we see historical recipes for mandrake-infused wine and henbane beer. By lowering inhibitions, relaxing the body, and potentiating the formulas they were mixed with, their powerful tropane alkaloids could induce a lust-filled frenzy.

Working with nightshades as aphrodisiacs shows us a very different side to these "dark and dangerous" plants, but in reality they are two sides to the same coin. Sex and death are connected, and when harnessed, these primal forces can open doorways to other realms and states of consciousness.

There are many reasons to engage in love magic, glamour, and sexuality in ritual. Spells to gain the attention and admiration of others are definitely part of this, but there is a deeper power to be discovered here. When we have love for ourselves, we stand fully in our power. This is easier said than done for many of us, myself included, and the journey to self-love is often a lifetime of daily reminders that we are worthy of that love. Every glamour is an act of self-affirmation, and what may look like narcissism to others can be an act of self-preservation. The dark and damaged things within us can stand in the way of self-actualization, and the plants in the nightshade family, as well as other poisonous and psychoactive herbs, can help us heal them.

Reasons to Use Love Magic

DRAWING MAGIC

- To attract love into your life
- To evoke self-love
- To attract the right partner
- To increase sexual receptivity
- To attract others
- To heal a broken heart, loneliness, or grief

GLAMOUR MAGIC

- To enhance people's perception of you through the aura, personal charms, and charisma
- To attract romantic attention, influence, and success
- For beautification rituals

COERCIVE LOVE MAGIC*

- To stir the passions of a specific person
- To gain the attention of a specific person

FIDELITY MAGIC

- To keep a lover faithful
- To cause a lover to return
- To keep a lover interested
- To bind a wandering lover

APHRODISIA

- To create feelings of lust and arousal
- To gain the attention of a suitor
- To intensify pleasure with a partner
- To rekindle the fires of passion
- To restore or enhance sexual nature, potency, and receptivity

SEX MAGIC

- To raise and direct energy
- To enter trance and communicate with spirits
- To connect with partners
- To heal trauma

*As noted earlier, coercive magic is potentially malefic.

Changing Perspectives

Please note that the following sections speak generally about sexual trauma. If this is a triggering subject for you, I encourage you to skip ahead to the section "Bringing Phytognosis to Other Modalities" on page 78.

Guilt and shame surrounding sexuality are prevalent. We are taught that sex is dirty, and that being or wanting to be sexual makes us dirty, and even more so if we don't fit in to society's sexual norm. The nightshade family is ready to help us break these limiting beliefs to pieces, using their bones to fertilize our gardens. Working with aphrodisiacs can lower our inhibitions and help us reconnect with this primal part of ourselves.

Belladonna, datura, henbane, and mandrake can help us through some of the shadow work that comes with learning to love ourselves. Their baneful nature connects them to shadow work and their aphrodisiac effects bring in the Venusian influence making them especially helpful for shadow work of a heart-related nature. Shadow work is uncomfortable. It requires us to intentionally go to all of the places within ourselves where we don't want to go, to look at the parts of ourselves that we don't want to see, and to acknowledge the damage in the places we don't think we need to heal. These baneful allies are not afraid to lead us into our own darkness, knowing that we will emerge changed for the better. Even on subtle levels, these plants are capable of inducing dramatic changes in our thought patterns, which is the first step to growth.

Healing Trauma

Trauma comes in many forms and can manifest differently for everyone. Everyone's definition of trauma is different, but if an experience felt traumatic to you, then it was trauma. We can become desensitized over time; we can begin to think that carrying trauma is normal, or that we deserved to have it happen to us, or that there is nothing we can do to change how we feel about it. Working with power plants, specifically nightshades, can help us separate ourselves from trauma so that we can get a new perspective on it.

These plants remind us that we are powerful, and that we do not have to accept anything that is not right for us. They help ground us, open us to the spirit world, and take us back to a primal place, deep in the shadows of the subconscious, where we fight our most difficult battles. Working with nightshades in ritual, whether as flower essences, herbal charms, infused oils, or other preparations, is like being in the VIP section, surrounded by bouncers. Theses plants will kill for us. They will fight for us. They will hold space for us when we need them to, pushing away everything that stands against us and reminding us that we are the most powerful force of all.

Opening the Heart

Love can feel like a battle, and sometimes we need to put on our armor and fight for ourselves. Other times we need to be more nurturing and gentle. Nightshades have gotten so much bad publicity over the years, but that is part of their charm. They can be dark, deadly, and sinister, but they are also great healers and loving teachers. Their family name, Solanaceae, derives from a Latin term meaning "to soothe," and medicinally they are analgesic (pain relieving) and soporific (sleep inducing). They can take away pain, take away memory, and send us into the deepest of sleep.

Working with these plants on a regular basis can sometimes leave us feeling closed off or isolated, or like we're being followed by a dark cloud. That is just part of who they are—it is their Saturnian nature. Sometimes we need this closed-off-ness to protect a damaged heart from further trauma while we heal or to renegotiate the boundaries in our life. At some point, however, we have to come back from this place and open ourselves up.

This is the path of balance. Healing comes from going into the darkness and then stepping back out into the light. To balance the heaviness that can come with some of the more baneful allies, we can seek the help of other magical heart healers and aphrodisiacs.

Herbs that strengthen and support the heart both physically and energetically, as well as those that create feelings of warmth and well-being, are perfect for this. My favorite heart-opening herbs are foxglove (flower essence), hawthorn berry, cacao, rose, and raspberry.

Standing in Your Power

Beyond healing, there is so much life to be lived! Even at a micro-dose level, most psychoactive plants and fungi have aphrodisiac effects or intoxicating effects that are well suited for amorous pursuits. Aphrodisiacs raise our vibration, open our hearts, bring warmth and light to our bodies, and enhance our sense of connectedness to others.

Aphrodisiacs don't always have to be about sex with a partner. They don't have to be about sex at all. Many aphrodisiacs are stimulating, warming, relaxing, and euphoric. These are all different energetic states that can help us better transmit a specific energy for magical intention. Initiating aphrodisiac states of consciousness while performing rituals, meditating, or chanting affirmations is an effective way to raise energy to direct toward a specific purpose.

Just allowing this energy to flow through you and radiating the love and warmth you are receiving outward is a powerful act that can have transformative effects on your life. Sending out energy and raising your vibration in this way is also one of the most effective ways to attract desirable things into your life. Attraction, abundance, and prosperity are all Venusian themes and are aligned with this energy. When we begin to live from a place of self-love, our power to attract and create becomes limitless.

Venusian Formulas for Personal Empowerment

The art of making potions, specifically love potions and charms of seduction, falls in the realm of Venus. The *ars veneris*, or art of Venus, as it was once known, was considered a type of malefic magic, an occult poisoning of the body and mind of another person in order to seduce them. The term *veneficium*, poison magic, comes from the same root word as *veneris*, and poison magic and love magic were seen to be closely related in ancient Rome.

> In the time of the Roman Empire, love potions or aquae amatrices (lover's waters) were highly sought after. The best of these came from Thessaly (a region of Greece) and had profound stupefying and arousing effects. Because most of their ingredients were grown in pleasure gardens, most of these magic potions were under the aegis of Venus.

Unfortunately, only a very few of these potions have come down to us. Most appear to have consisted of wine, to which various herbs, plant juices, roots and resins were added. Many of the active ingredients were nightshades. Opium, hemp, basil and cinnamon were also common ingredients. (Rätsch and Müller-Ebeling 2005, 19)

The knowledge of plants and their uses in magic and medicine was the domain of the goddess Venus. This included knowledge of poisonous plants as well. Like the goddess herself, Nature holds the power to give life and take it away. Venus, as an archetype for understanding numinous forces, has a dualistic nature. She is a goddess of infinite beauty and grace, but also a bloodthirsty and relentless she-demon. Both have great wisdom and power to share, and this is the crooked path of the witch, for whom Venus is also patron.

Venusberg (Venus Mountain) was the site of the medieval witches' Sabbath in Europe, and Venus was queen of its proceedings. In this role, Venus is the Witch Queen. She is a patron of herbal knowledge and healing with nature. She is also the face of death, the cold hand pushing us to confront our own darkness. Working with this aspect of the witch goddess, as a tutelary spirit in wortcunning has been central in my personal practice.

Like the goddess Venus and her counterparts, Venusian magic can be either innocent and amorous or malefic and manipulative. The following formulas encompass both light and dark aspects of Venusian workings, and like all magical workings they can be put to a spectrum of magical intentions.

Bend Over Oil

- Dried herbs: bergamot, calamus root, and licorice root
- Carrier oil
- Essential oils: bergamot, calamus root, and licorice root
- A pinch of damiana, cubeb berries, or grains of paradise

Create a base oil by infusing equal parts of the dried herbs in carrier oil for 3 weeks. Strain out the plant material and add the essential oils. Before bottling, add a pinch of damiana, cubeb berries, or grains of paradise.

Use this oil to anoint your body when in the presence of those whose will you wish to bend.

Spicy Love Dusting Powder

All the herbs should be in dried form.

- ❧ Cayenne pepper
- ❧ Cinnamon
- ❧ Datura leaves
- ❧ Ginger
- ❧ Grains of paradise

Powder equal parts of all the herbs in a mortar and pestle. Use the resulting powder to dust the bedroom, clothing, or draw Venusian symbols. Avoid getting in the eyes or sensitive areas.

Jezebel Oil

Jezebel, a Phoenician princess in the ninth century BCE, married King Ahab of Israel. She is vilified in the Old Testament for persuading the king to worship the god Baal, a pagan nature deity. All sorts of cruel and tyrannical acts are attributed to her. She became the model for the "wicked woman," a patriarchal concept used in Abrahamic religion to demonize strong and independent women. Jezebel was the embodiment of cruelty, greed, and vanity, according to . . . men. On the other hand, she was a powerful woman acting with sovereignty, opulence, and charisma. She also stayed true to the beliefs of her people and brought pagan religion back to Israel for a time. She represents the old gods and is an enchantress in her own right.

The herb known as Jezebel root comes from one of five species of Louisiana iris. Its use in magic derives from hoodoo and African American folk practice (which has influenced American folk magic in general). Jezebel root is traditionally used to attract a wealthy and generous male lover. It also has a dark and manipulative side, not only attracting but dominating this gentleman. Great for BDSM!

The Curse of Jezebel is a notorious working using the whole root. It is a curse of vengeance, destruction, and righteous anger.

Jezebel oil is one of my favorite formulas because of everything it represents. If your income relies on you being appealing to the carnal appetites of others, it is a powerful oil to wear. Sex workers can use it to attract wealthy clients who want to spend money. Dancers, escorts, drag queens, servers, and bartenders can all use this oil to boost their charisma and nerve. Creatures of the night, they use the shadows to their advantage to bring fantasy to life.

If you are looking for a sugar daddy or wanting to dominate your man in the bedroom, this sweet and dusky oil will enhance your allure and sexual prowess. Jezebel root itself has an affinity with gay men, with similar properties to Queen Elizabeth root. It can be used for anything from love spells to hookups.

This is my own formula for Jezebel oil, using the root from the species Iris fulva. It has a musky, multilayered fragrance that is sweet with hints of rose, benzoin, spikenard, and honey.

- Ashwagandha
- Benzoin resinoid
- Deer's tongue
- Honey
- Jasmine essential oil
- Jezebel root
- Mandrake root or leaves (depending on availability)
- Orris root
- Rose fragrance oil

- Spikenard essential oil
- Carrier oil

Infuse the herbs in the oil, then strain out the solid matter and bottle the oil. My personal Jezebel oil is an on-going infusion that grows more concentrated over time. The minimum time for an oil infusion of this nature is 3 to 4 weeks and can be started on a Friday in the hour of Venus. There are no specific amounts for the plant material or essential oils that can be added based on availability and personal preference regarding which scents are most pleasing to you. I like to keep a larger "mother" bottle containing the plant material adding more herbs and essential oils as needed. Smaller working bottles can be filled with oil that has been strained.

Euphoric Kava Infusion

*Kava (*Piper methysticum*) is calming and euphoric, with sensory-enhancing qualities. This recipe makes enough for one person.*

- 2–4 tablespoons (7–14 grams) kava root powder
- 450 ml water
- Cream or full-fat coconut milk (helps with absorption)
- Cinnamon
- Nutmeg

Place the powdered kava root in a clean glass jar and pour boiling water over it. Cover and let steep for 8 to 12 hours. Strain, using cheesecloth and squeezing out all the liquid. Add cream or coconut milk and cinnamon and nutmeg. Serve warm or cold.

Sip kava slowly, and drink until you begin to notice your mouth become numb and tingly, then stop drinking and what around 20 minutes to determine if you need to drink more. Over time, the amount of kava you need to feel its effects decreases.

※

Rose Chain-Breaker

If memory serves me right, I learned about the basis forformula from Harold Roth, author of The Witching Herbs *(2017) and adapted it. Its original intention is to break through Venusian enchantments and illusions by using the apple cider vinegar to "sour" the Venusian energies. The formula smells of dusky rose, chthonic and nocturnal in nature. It can be used in break-up spells, rituals to heal a broken heart, and situations when love has died and it is time to move on.*

- ❧ 1 dozen red roses
- ❧ Apple cider vinegar
- ❧ Dried pomegranate pieces
- ❧ Red wine
- ❧ Jasmine essential oil
- ❧ Lotus fragrance oil
- ❧ Rose hydrosol, rose fragrance oil, or rose otto

Pull the heads off the roses and place them in a mason jar. Cover halfway with apple cider vinegar, then add the pomegranate pieces and fill the rest of the jar with red wine. Allow this to infuse for 3 days, then strain out the plant material and add the jasmine and lotus oils and rose hydrosol. Use this formula in ritual baths and to anoint the body.

Aphrodisiac Tea/Smoke Blend

- ❧ 1 part damiana
- ❧ 1 part rose petals
- ❧ ½ part passion flower
- ❧ ⅛ part vanilla bean

Grind the herbs to a uniform consistency. Brew 1 to 2 tablespoons per cup of water or smoke your desired amount.

If you're making this formula into a tea blend, I suggest adding

1 to 2 tablespoons of cacao powder to the entire mixture and a pinch of powdered sugar and honey to each cup when it's brewing.

✿

Damiana-Infused Wine

Damiana adds its stimulating and aphrodisiac affects to the wine, along with its complementary warm flavor. Traditional mulling spices could be added for more flavor, if desired.

- 1 bottle red wine
- ½ ounce damiana
- 2 cinnamon sticks

Pour the wine into a saucepan and add the cinnamon sticks and damiana. Bring to a simmer over low heat, cover, and let simmer for 25 minutes. Serve the wine warm or chilled.

SHADOW WORK

Shadow work has become something of a trend. That's not to invalidate those who are doing the work. Many people are being drawn to shadow work right now because of what is going on in our society, on both a domestic and global scale, but in reality we are all doing shadow work in some form or another. Human consciousness is changing; we are becoming more than what we were. Though this change will eventually have positive results, right now, in the midst of it, we see nothing but chaos, turmoil, and upheaval. Individually, globally, and cosmically, we are purging the restrictions that have been put upon us, embracing the hidden parts of ourselves, and coming together in ways we never thought possible.

Shadow work is about finding power in our dark side. It is a exploration of our inner darkness for healing, for empowerment, and to release that which does not serve. It is about embracing the parts of ourselves that society has told us are taboo. We do not seek to become our shadow; it is already part of us. And it doesn't define us any more than our more socially acceptable qualities do.

Shadow work is inner work, done in the darkness, done alone. The shadow is not just the negative, repressed, ignored, and shameful parts of ourselves. It is the part of us that tells us we must be perfect, that we must attain success at all costs, that we are not good enough. It is good at disguising itself as desirable qualities. Shadow aspects occur when we have not healed or processed painful emotions or when we ignore our inner voice. The self becomes fragmented, and these fragments act against each other. Shadow work teaches us not only to embrace but to train these parts of ourselves to work in our favor.

Shadow work is about healing trauma. It is about finding the root of the bullshit in our lives and, instead of trying to tear it out, cultivating that part of ourselves into something beautiful. Those roots are all feeding the same tree, and we need the decaying matter for our soil as much as we need the sunlight for our leaves. Like the earth beneath our feet, the shadow is where we all come from and where we all long to return. It is the dark primordial womb of the mother.

Baneful herbs and poisonous plants have a special affinity for shadow work. This is because they are the shadow of the plant world. Their connection to death, danger, sex, and intoxication makes them knowledgeable teachers when it comes to facing those very things, which are so often the source of our own shadows. On an energetic level, poisonous plants are very powerful.

All baneful herbs are predisposed to shadow work in general, but they also have their individual attributes. These include:

- ✦ Purging stagnant energy
- ✦ Cutting cords with attachments that are draining your energy (energetic parasites)
- ✦ Healing trauma (conscious and unconscious)
- ✦ Bringing things to the surface to be consciously processed
- ✦ Integrating and facilitating transformative experiences

✦ Creating new and healthy boundaries

✦ Journeying to meet the shadow

✦ Facing death, mortality, and grief

✦ Healing shame around issues of sex, submission, or dominance

✦ Healing from religious trauma

✦ Recovering from addiction, abuse, or PTSD

ঞ *Embracing the Shadow Meditation*

This is a very simple meditation that anyone can do, and it is immediately effective. You can choose a poison plant ally to help with the shadow work. Flower essences work well; they really shine in the mental and emotional realm. Sit in a comfortable position for this meditation. Slightly reclined is fine. Just make sure you can get your arms around yourself. Begin with the intention to connect with your shadow. Consume your plant material mindfully, holding your intention.

Focus on your breathing. Deep breath in, deep breath out. Don't force it; get into a comfortable rhythm.

Close your eyes. Visualize the plant material within you. See the plant spirit energy emanating off it as an emerald green color within your body. Every time you breathe in, picture this green energy creeping out a little farther, spreading through your entire body.

Once you are completely relaxed and full of the plant's energy, turn your attention to your surroundings. Visualize yourself outside in a natural place. It is nighttime.

Begin to casually explore your surroundings, following whatever path your feet choose. Eventually you find a stream or waterfall or hear the sound of water. Follow it to a reflective pool. Or maybe you find an antique mirror overgrown with ivy.

You catch a glimpse of yourself in the pool or mirror. It is you, but not you. This version of yourself is dark and twisted, giving you a sense of strangeness. You don't recognize the familiar face looking back at you. Take time to study the reflection. This is your shadow. There may be a conversation or perhaps a silent exchange between you. As the time passes, the reflection begins to slowly emerge from the reflective surface until your shadow self is standing in front of you.

As you stand facing your shadow self, continue to take deep breaths. Picture that green light of your plant spirit ally shining out from your heart as you embrace your shadow self. This should feel uncomfortable at first. While you do this, take your physical arms and wrap them around yourself as tightly as you can, giving yourself a big hug. Sit like this for a while, taking deep breaths, and imagine that green light growing brighter. This light feeds you and your shadow, strengthening your connection and bringing you closer together. The green light increases until it is too bright to see, at which point you begin to return to waking consciousness.

It takes a long time to really understand and embrace your shadow, but this simple act of self-love is extremely cathartic. The plant spirit ally helps you connect with the shadow on a vibrational level so that both of you benefit from this exercise.

Many people find themselves overwhelmed with emotion when performing this exercise. Our society lacked human contact and affection before the COVID-19 pandemic, and now more than ever we need to feel that physical love. You can perform this exercise regularly as part of your self-care regimen.

BRINGING PHYTOGNOSIS TO OTHER MODALITIES

One of the aspects of the poison path as a spiritual practice is identifying and transmuting spiritual toxins that overtime can have a detrimental influence on our well-being and growth as individuals. Whether it is fear, shame, or an unhealthy behavioral pattern we can apply these practices and philosophies to help move these blockages and transform them into a source of strength. We can tap into the power of poison plant allies to get support and understanding for the demons that we are facing. For example, we can work with the spirit of belladonna to help with issues of control, self-image, and love. Datura can help us with deeply rooted fears, trauma, and toxic behaviors. We can even call upon the help of other mind-body-altering plants to help facilitate this process on a physical level to help facilitate this process energetically and spiritually. By altering the chemistry of the body and mind as we employ these practices we are taking a multifaceted approach to loosening the hold these thought patterns and behaviors may have on us.

Plants can be used in conjunction with other wellness practices to enhance the effects of both. You can incorporate a plant for its supportive or medicinal effects, for its psychoactive quality, or to work with it on an energetic or spiritual level. Often all three aspects come into play, as we receive all these benefits from the plants whether we are using them for only mundane or only spiritual uses.

Plant medicine offers profound insight and healing through phytognosis. When we combine that with body work, meaning techniques that put us in touch with the physical body, these effects become pronounced. Using various techniques of energy work, breathing, or body postures, we can begin to influence the direction and flow of our plant spirit work.

Other techniques of meditation and trance work can also benefit from or expand upon phytognosis.

Yoga and other movement based practices are enhanced with the incorporation of plant spirit medicine. Cannabis yoga is the perfect example of this, in which participants consume cannabis before beginning their practice. While not technically a poisonous plant, cannabis does have mind-altering effects and it has been demonized because of those effects in much the same way that more deadly plants have been demonized. By incorporating plants like cannabis, blue lotus, kava, or damiana into these practices we are able to better get in touch with our bodies, and let go of thoughts and emotions that stand in our way. Through the relaxing and euphoric effects of these plant allies we are able to deepen our yoga practice, which allows for more profound inner work. By focusing on the movement of the body and breath in combination with plant medicine we are able to better access areas that need to be processed.

Shamanic postures are used to travel to other worlds and generate altered states. Shamanic body postures are similar to yoga postures in the sense that they allow us to access altered states of consciousness more efficiently. Shamanic body postures can be used for various purposes from divination to otherworld travel. In combination with plant spirit allies we are able to use these postures to access specific parts of the spirit world and communicate with spirit allies, ancestors, and deities to assist us in our pursuits.

Hand positions or mudras can help us focus our energy when we are working with plant spirit allies.

Drumming enhances the effects of plants. It facilitates trance states and healing and moves energy.

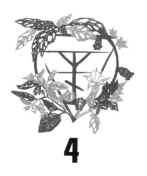

4

Dark Herbalism

Walking through the Shadow World

*W*hen we're going on an important journey to a place we've never been before, to a place that is unfamiliar or scary, it helps to have a guide—someone who has made this journey before. The same can be said for our spiritual journeys and journeys of healing and transformation. While we can turn to many healing and tonic herbs for light, comfort, and support during times of darkness, we also can find tremendous power and enlightenment when we enlist the help of baneful herbs.

I use the term *dark herbalism* in recognition of the inherent difference in plants that have these qualities. The manner in which they derive or manifest their "dark" properties tells us a lot about their occult properties. Are they poisonous or invasive? Physically dangerous? Connected to the dead? Carnivorous plants, thorns and brambles, night-blooming flowers—these, too, also occupy a space in the dark pharmacopoeia. Dark herbalism appreciates and respects the sinister and trepidatious qualities of plants and their ability to heal in different ways. It explores the unexplored parts of nature and works with forces not typically sought out willingly. It is not all about being spooky; it seeks to decipher what attracts us to or repels us from certain things and the emotions and energies they awaken within us.

ALLIES OF DARKNESS

Baneful herbs have special qualities that set them apart from those considered benign or beneficial. They are just as healing as their innocuous counterparts, but their healing is of a different sort. Think of them as "wounded healers": They have been into battle; they have seen things and done things. Some have been used historically for murder, malice, and all sorts of manipulation. These plants have been marked by the ways in which humans have used (or abused) them. By connecting with them as allies, we can transform that human darkness, or maleficia, that surrounds them, just as they can help us transform the darkness within ourselves.

Dark Herbalism

Plants are not good or evil, but like all forces of nature, they are powerful. Sometimes that power makes them threatening to humans. Dark herbalism seeks to harness that power, seeking out the plants that have been deemed taboo, dangerous, toxic, pernicious, noxious, invasive, and/or sepulchral. Nature is not black or white; it is green. A plant's characteristics and virtues are all filtered through the lens of our own perception. Plant life begins in darkness, as a seed, and it is from the darkness of the soil that the plant continues to draw nourishment. Most plants also filter sunlight to create energy, and they are all influenced by the seasons. In other words, plants (and humans) get what they need to thrive from both the fertile darkness and the vitalizing light. Dark herbalism considers light and dark as an analogy for the dual facets of a being's energy or spirit, understanding that there are many steps in between and that their nature is not fixed.

It is in exploring the shadows, the dark forest, and the hidden or occult part of nature that we find some of the greatest wisdom. It is also here, in the shadow of the tree of life, that we can experience profound healing. In looking at some of the stories these plants tell, we learn that the mythical monsters and witches meant to scare people away from these plants are, in reality, guardians and teachers of deeper wisdom.

Healing with Poison

The word *baneful* derives from Old English, meaning something capable of causing harm. There are lots of ways plants can cause us harm, and that is not limited to the many physical wounds they can inflict. Banefulness is an ominous quality attributed to plants that are capable of more than healing. When they are a threat or nuisance to agricultural crops, a danger to animals or humans, uncontrollable, invasive, or unwanted, they take on an adversarial nature in their folklore, but they are no villains. Their "baneful" qualities are reflections of our own baneful qualities: our fear, our desire to control and manipulate, our desire to destroy.

This is the reason why these plants are so helpful for shadow work, arduous transitions, and the other difficult experiences that we humans encounter. They are connected in sympathetic and intimate ways to many of the emotions, energies, and obstacles that we face. By working with baneful herbs, we can heal our relationship with our self, and in turn our connection to the natural world.

Baneful plants are warriors, dangerous to the unknowing and terrible to behold. They are the guides of the dead, soothing and appeasing their spirits. They are the allies of the cunning sorcerer who seduces and destroys. They are the herbs of the seer, traveler of worlds, who has been to the otherworld and returned changed. Powerful both medicinally and magically, these herbs possess qualities and virtues that cause people to fear them. Yet it is in their "baneful" nature that their power and their medicine lie.

It could be said that all plants have a dualistic nature, with both dark and light aspects, just like people. Elder, for example, is a common medicinal herb, yet the elder tree is said to be home to devils and witches and a gateway to the spirit world. Sunny, cheerful dandelion is another; though edible and broadly useful in medicine, it can also be used to summon spirits and connect with ancestors. It is in plants' hidden or dark side that some of their most interesting characteristics, and those that offer the most profound results, can be found.

The Saturnian Nature

Not all baneful herbs are poisonous, but all poisonous plants have a baneful quality. All poisonous plants are ruled by Saturn (though they often exhibit other planetary and elemental qualities as well). That said, not all herbs ruled by Saturn are poisonous; arnica, Solomon's seal, and comfrey are good examples of Saturnian plants that are not poisonous. Saturnian herbs tend to grow in wasteland, on decomposing material. They tend to have tiny white flowers and large earthy roots. Though their flowers are generally unscented, the plants themselves may have a fetid odor or smell like decomposing meat. That said, not all Saturnian herbs will share all these qualities.

Medicinally, Saturnian herbs are astringent, cold, drying, soporific (sedative), and effective at strengthening and healing bones and connective tissue. They slow and cool things down.

Metaphysically, Saturnian herbs relate to things like structure, foundation, time, restriction, inversion, past trauma, earth, groundedness and heaviness, boundaries, and limits (strengthening and going beyond them).

In medieval lore, Saturn was associated with witches (and all other things malefic). Yet he was a very ancient agricultural deity before he gained his darker connotations. Looking at his mythology, we see connections between this figure, various horned gods, and the Devil. He is said to have been the ruler of the Saturnian golden age, the time before the Olympian gods (Michael 2021).

Saturn's herbs are used in hexing, binding, banishing, protection, spirit communication, summoning spirits, necromancy, underworld travel, cutting cords, creating stronger boundaries, shadow work, secrecy, hiding and revealing hidden things, and spirit pacts.

Accessing Vibrational Energy

We can access a plant's spirit medicine through the use of vibrational remedies, charms, and amulets. Through this energetic connection, the herbs affect us on a mental, emotional, or spiritual level.

Below is a list of well-known baneful herbs and some of their vibrational qualities. The idea that poisonous plants can heal us is a strange one. However, the "poisonous" nature of a plant lies in the dosage. When a so-called poisonous plant is used in small dosages, the effects are much different and medically useful. The same principle becomes even more true when we are talking about vibrational remedies like homeopathic preparations and flower essences. A plant acts differently in these infinitesimally small dosages, and its energetic effects are amplified. For these reasons, vibrational remedies are a safe way of obtaining the benefits from these toxic plants.

FOXGLOVE: THE PROTECTOR

- Affects the heart and emotional body, filling us with loving vibrations
- Helps with self-love and overcoming feelings of loneliness and abandonment
- Eases heart conditions, angina, apprehension and anxiety about the future, and fear of death; supports us in letting go of remorse or guilt
- Calms an overworked mind and internal anxieties
- Used in homeopathic doses to treat a slow heartbeat
- Strengthens the heart, treating heart failure and irregularities
- Calms emotions related to relationship trauma
- Eases feelings of vulnerability
- Protects the heart and feelings

MONKSHOOD: THE HERMIT

- Facilitates introspection, inner reality, and realignment with the self
- Stabilizes the emotional body after trauma
- Offers support for fear, shock, anxiety, chronic difficulties, or past/childhood traumas

- Supports us in breaking past indoctrination and dogma
- Cultivates qualities of spiritual leadership and integrity
- Supports psychic ability and a sense of identity/authentic self

DATURA (D. STRAMONIUM): THE TRICKSTER/SHAMAN

- Supports us in dealing with the process of death and the fear of dying; helps with grief and mourning
- Brings clarity and insight to dreams
- Confers strength in confronting fears and anxiety
- Calms restlessness, helps dispel nightmares, delusions, night terrors
- Purges unwanted energies and harmful influences; removes attachments
- Brings a change of perspective, helping us through periods of transformation

POISON HEMLOCK: THE BLADE

- Offers release from what is holding you back or keeping you captive
- Helps us reclaim personal power through voice
- Helps with exhaustion and loss of interest
- Balances extreme sexual excitement and releases suppressed sexuality
- Releases emotional paralysis caused by fear
- Helps ease transitions
- Detoxifies the emotional body

DEADLY NIGHTSHADE: THE FURY

- Facilitates understanding of death, fate, spirituality, and sexuality
- Supports us in cutting energetic cords and releasing harmful attachments to people and the past
- Helps calm anger and agitation
- Helps those who are hypersensitive to stimuli
- Brings clarity so we can see through illusions and cut ties
- Supports us in taking back personal power

PLANTAE INFERNUM:
THE DARK SIDE OF NATURE

Nature has many fantastic and sometimes destructive powers. Our perception of these powers is filtered through our human experience. From our point of view, natural events like floods, thunderstorms, and hail are a threat, and so we perceive these forces differently than we do things like sunlight, the smell of flowers, and the fertility of the land. While all aspects of nature can be beneficial or detrimental under the right circumstances, and depending on the perspective, certain forces are so vast that they lie beyond our understanding; we call them mysterious and "dark."

We describe things in terms of dark and light because it gives us a sense of their nature—from *our* perspective. Lightning does not care what or who it strikes, and fire will consume all that it can, but from our perspective being struck by lightning or burned by fire is generally a bad thing. That is *not* to say that all "dark" things are dangerous or bad—quite the opposite. We are talking here about primal forces. Humans naturally like to categorize all the aspects of the world in order to have a reference point for where they fit in the grand scheme of things, and the way that we do this tells us more about ourselves and the forces we are encountering than about any moral direction they might have.

Darkness is not just the absence of light, it is the medium in which light exists. Without darkness, light has no matrix to graft itself to. Before illumination, darkness holds infinite potential.

This concept cannot be more evident than in the plant world. We categorize plants as medicinal, toxic, poisonous, agricultural, ornamental, invasive, and more, and these labels are largely based on whether or not a plant is beneficial for commercial agriculture. Some plants are grown for profit or to feed one of our modern addictions; the others are largely demonized and vilified.

The relationship between humans and plants is so important. It is one of our oldest and longest-lasting relationships, and plants are some of our greatest allies. They build our homes and nourish our bodies. Countless healing and medicinal plants are capable of helping us in many ways, and we have a more familiar relationship with these socially acceptable plants. Yet it is in relationships with the unfamiliar that we can find the most growth and understanding. Forming a relationship with the unwanted and ostracized members of the plant kingdom, including weeds, invasives, and poisonous plants, can teach us much about ourselves and the world around us. It is here that we can heal ourselves, but more importantly, we can heal our relationship with the natural world.

A plant's history and lore give us clues to its potential applications in magical practice. The relationship a plant has had with humans and how we describe that relationship tells us about the characteristics of the plant's spirit. It is difficult to find a plant (among those we have discovered) that doesn't have some kind of folklore, superstition, or ritual use attached to it. Some plants have an extensive body of folklore and magical correspondences, while others may have only one or two qualities that have been recorded.

Some plants have a particularly malevolent or even diabolical reputation. They are believed to be home to evil spirits or even tended to by the Devil himself.* These infernal plants are capable of summoning spirits, delivering death, and creating all manner of maleficia. Much of the superstition and vilification regarding these plants leads to deeper wisdom and in many cases Indigenous or folk knowledge that Western church authorities attempted to eradicate.

Many of these plants have been used (and regulated) for their aphrodisiac, psychoactive, and poisonous properties. Plants capable of altering consciousness and promoting independent spiritual connection have

---

*You could write an entire book (see the bibliography) just on plants with a common name referring to the Devil. This is the folkloric Devil, the wild adversary in nature, connected to the many-horned gods. He is not an evil spirit but a trickster, wild and untamable.

always been a threat to institutionalized religion and called the work of the Devil. The term *entheogen* literally translates as "to generate the divine within," and these mind-altering plants and fungi, through their phytochemistry, are capable of inducing spiritual and magical experiences when applied in a ritual setting. These plants often have a long history of ceremonial use and are still revered by Indigenous people in different parts of the world today. Psilocybin mushrooms, ayahuasca brews, cannabis, and tobacco have all been used entheogenically by people for spiritual purposes for millennia. These were the herbs burned in sacred temple incense and infused into ceremonial drinks taken to heal and connect the community.

Entheogen is a very broad term, and there are many different states of consciousness, and plants that are capable of enhancing those different states. There are also many different ways to access and apply these states, whether for divination, dreamwork, spirit communication, and so on. Psychedelic historian Thomas Hatsis distinguishes these nuances with terms like *pythiagen, oneirogen,* and *mystheogen* in his book *Psychedelic Mystery Traditions*. These distinctions describe which particular way an entheogen is being employed, and many can be used in a variety of different ways. *Pythiagens* are entheogens used for divinatory purposes. *Oneirogens* are entheogens employed for their dream-inducing effects, and *mystheogens* are entheogens used in a magical capacity as part of a ritual.

While all these experiences can be considered divine—that is, relating to the spirit world—there are certain times when they can take on a darker theme. Traveling to the underworld for ancestral knowledge or to retrieve healing, exploring the shadow, connecting with infernal spirits, and working with deities associated with primal forces like death and magic are not celestially oriented in the same manner as other practices. Instead of climbing the world tree, we descend into its roots. The baneful plants that help us in this endeavor act as emissaries, helping us to connect with the beings that dwell there. They are *chthonigens,* plants of the underworld.

There are a wide variety of ways to work with herbs in ritual for their occult virtues, and that does not always mean ingesting them. Some of these plants are poisonous and should be worked with only under certain circumstances. Using these herbs in charms, fetishes, and vibrational remedies, for example, are safe ways to incorporate their spirits into our magic. It is important that you understand what herbs are safe to work with, and how to do so, before you start experimenting.

THE DEVIL'S GARDEN: EMBRACING ADVERSARY AS ALLY

Humans have long associated the untamable and dangerous wilderness with malevolent forces. Dark forests, marshy wastelands, and other places that humans tend to avoid have a threatening aura and have been said to be inhabited by ghosts and monsters of all sorts. The Devil is said to lurk between the rows of corn, inside the roots of the elder tree, and throughout the haunted wilderness.

Just as we see in the names of uncommon geological formations (Devil's Stairway, Devil's Backbone, Devil's Tower), which are often the sacred sites of Indigenous peoples, for a plant the name *devil's (fill in the blank)* signifies something out of the ordinary or beyond human control. Many of the plants that share this nomenclature are sacred to Indigenous peoples, carry shamanic importance, and are featured in local mythology. They also have strong associations with magic, witchcraft, and sorcery.

> Speaking generally, trees, plants and herbs of ill omen may be placed in the category of plants of the Devil, and amongst them must be included such as have the reputation of being accursed, enchanted, unlucky, and sorrowful. Plants dedicated to Hecate, the Grecian goddess of Hell who presided over magic and enchantments, as well as those made use of by her daughters, Medea and Circe, in their sorceries were all satanic. The spells of wizards, magicians, witches, and others who were acquainted with the black art were all made

in name with of the Devil. Thus, all herbs and plants employed by them became veritable herbs of the Devil. (Folkard 1884, 55)

The term *devil's garden* can denote many things: a physical space set aside and left to grow wild, a metaphor for all feared and hated plants, or a location beyond time and space where we can go to retrieve knowledge and medicine from our plant allies.

Certain plants evoke strong emotions within us: fear, awe, or uncertainty about their strangeness. Working with such plants can inspire an awakening. It allows us to open the gates to the underworld and explore the shadows within ourselves, not to banish or integrate them, but to befriend them, to nurture them, and to forge relationships with them. Plants like devil's eye, devil's bit, and devil's walking stick all have a unique story to tell. Considering the devil's garden as a category of plants that share this quality shows us how we can rework their adversarial qualities into exercises of personal power.

> *The association between certain plants and the Devil has therefore formed a natural linkage, one that has served to perpetuate the forbidding and wicked plant lore to a deeper degree, over time.*
>
> CORINNE BOYER, *PLANTS OF THE DEVIL*

There is a certain allure that these plants possess, one that simultaneously draws us in, but warns us of something potentially sinister that lies beyond. The transgressive act of seeking out that which is taboo or off limits offers potential for transformation via personal gnosis transmitted through the adversarial forces of nature. These adversarial figures appear throughout human myth and religion, outside of the norms of society, these vilified and feared entities are the allies of the witch and magical practitioner. Often seen as a scapegoat for societies' fears and repressed desires, these beings have much to teach us and the plants of the devil's garden are one means of connecting to their energies.

Trickster Spirits, Adversarial Allies, Horned Gods, and Sacrificed Deities

✦ Exist in many cultures and often play an adversarial role

✦ Can be ambivalent toward humans

✦ Share knowledge via sacrifice and transformation

✦ Tricksters are shapeshifters

✦ Prometheus, Lucifer, Loki, Coyote—these and other tricksters were punished for giving humans something that was originally in the possession of the gods. While feared and demonized, these mischievous entities were sympathetic to the difficulties faced by early humankind, and wanted to see us prosper. By putting their own well-being in jeopardy these "fallen ones" are attributed with giving us the very tools that we would use to create civilizations including the use of fire, the arts, and the sciences. It is through their sacrifice that we are where we are today.

✦ The Devil isn't the only one with horns: Pan, Dionysius, Baphomet, the Horned God, Cernunnos. Horns were also added to statues as symbols of wisdom and divinity, including images of the Old Testament figure Moses.

✦ Woodland spirits, fauns, satyrs, sylvan spirits, harvest gods, woodwose or wild men of the forest, or green men are all spirits associated with wildness, unbridled sexuality, and the untamable sides of ourselves that we are taught to keep hidden.

The Adversarial Spirit—The Green Devil

✦ Challenges us and our conceptions of reality, magical practice, and spirit work

✦ Sacrifice must be made to work with this spirit intimately

✦ Given offerings out of respect for the wild, giving back control to nature

✦ Sacrifices made to the land, shares of crops given to the Devil to ensure it wasn't spoiled

Everything in nature kills to survive, and this is something not lost on us despite the efforts of society to disconnect us from the natural world. Without our modern conveniences, availability of tools, resources, and shelter we would be left with the reality that most of us would not survive very long. Our supremacy over this world is an illusion, and the adversarial and wild spirits of nature seek to remind us of that. This is a concept that reminds us, especially green practitioners, to pay our respects to the primal powers of the natural world that will exist long after our time here as a species has ended.

Cain, the First Farmer

The biblical figure of Cain is said to have been cursed and banished by Yahweh, who preferred Cain's brother Abel's sacrifice of goats versus the harvest that Cain offered. Angered by this rejection, Cain murdered Abel and became one of the first adversarial spirits that would ally themselves with the arcane arts. Today, he is associated with witchcraft and vampirism and is honored as a patron of wort-cunning and the poison path.

Curiously, Cain is often known as the first farmer, and farmers are responsible for many of the folk names we have for plants—especially those adversarial green spirits that thwart cultivation efforts and earned themselves the name *devil*.

The Devil we speak of is not the red-cape-wearing Devil of cartoons nor the Satan of the Old Testament. This is a different Devil—the green Devil, the Devil of folklore. This Devil represents power, and as the green Devil, he can be found among adversarial plants, including those that are poisonous, invasive, difficult to kill, thorny, and more. These plants represent the wild and untamable wilderness. They are the powers that resist human control. We can tap into these powers for:

✦ Gnosis (knowledge)
✦ Healing through transformation and transmutation
✦ Protection from oppression and manipulation
✦ Personal power and rebellion against constructs
✦ Connecting to the spirits of the land
✦ Working with dark herbalism

The Devil's Acre

The *Devil's Acre* is traditionally a small plot of land left uncultivated—left to grow wild—as an offering to ensure good crops for the rest of a farm. Whatever grew there was said to belong to the Devil.

Today, anyone wanting to make such an offering would not need a full acre, of course. Even a small square of a garden or a corner of a homeowner's property is sufficient. You could build a cairn, using stones from the property, to serve as an altar for offerings. This can eventually become a place to connect with genii loci (land spirits), to access the spirit world, and to collect plants for ritual. The Devil's Acre is a reservoir of transgressive power, and while all things within its boundaries belong to the Old One, offerings can be made in exchange for herbs and other ingredients that can be found within its bounds. The things collected from this area, once paid for, make powerful ingredients for formulas and spell work and should only be collected under important circumstances with full understanding of whom you are collecting these items from. Every herb, root, stone, and soil collected from the Devil's Acre carries within it an implicit pact, and in exchange for a piece of its power somber and meaningful offerings must be made. These offerings will differ for each individual and the work at hand. Anything collected from this space for ritual must be paid for with a sacrifice; the greater the gift, the greater the return.

The Devil's Due

The Devil's Due is a means of maintaining the connection between practitioner, the Land, and their magical practice through feeding the Devil's Acre. By depositing your ritual remains including ashes of incense, poppets, root fetishes, and other by-products of the witches' arte, you forge a powerful link to the spirits of the land.

To maintain the power, presence, and personal connection to the Devil's Acre, regular offerings should be made to infuse your work with the potency of the Green Devil; this is called the Devil's Due, which pays respect to the agency behind your magical workings. Collect an offering for the green Devil, calling him into all of your workings by doing so. The following can be ritually collected and later deposited in the Devil's Acre or other wild place:

- ✦ A leaf or flower plucked from every plant in the garden
- ✦ Ritual ashes from incense, burned petitions, or ritual fires
- ✦ A drop of every potion, tincture, or formula used in a ritual

Call upon the Green Devil for protection, personal agency, sovereignty, rebellion, occult pursuits, and pact making.

THE POISON ALLURE:
POWER PLANTS FOR MEDICINE AND MAGIC

Why work with poisonous plants at all? Poisonous doesn't always mean deadly, though it certainly can when it comes to some of the more dangerous plants like hemlock and aconite. Some plants won't kill you but can give you uncomfortable symptoms and even put you in the hospital. On one end of the spectrum we find irritating plants like poison ivy, which are considered "poisonous" because they are bothersome to humans. On the opposite end of the spectrum are plants like gympie-gympie (a.k.a. suicide plant), which is native to Australia. This plant's leaves are covered in stinging hairs that cause such intense pain people have killed themselves to make it stop. So, "poisonous" can mean very different things, and as we've noted previously, the poison is all in the dosage. The same qualities that make an herb poisonous are also what make it medicinal, whether that's in minute doses, in vibrational remedies, or in spirit medicine.

That said, some plants are so dangerous that they are best appreciated from afar. Don't put yourself in harm's way. There are plants that can blind you, burn you, and scar you for life. Poison is potency.

We seek to work with poisonous plants for different reasons. As noted earlier, poison magic, or veneficium, has long been part of the repertoire of the witch. Thanks to this association, many poisonous plants are often intimately connected with the practice of witchcraft and its associated spirits.

These baneful herbs also have healing qualities, albeit of a different sort than traditional medicinal plants. While medicinal tonic herbs tend to be more projective with their energy, poisonous plants are more restrictive. This is in part due to their Saturnian nature, being cold and soporific, they remove heat and inflammation, cause sleep, and when taken in excess can slow respiration and heart rate. This is both where their value as medicinal herbs lies but also their potential as poisons. Again, the harmful nature of these herbs are based on their application in a highly individualized situation, and their effects a matter of dosage. Yet a plant's phytotoxins—the chemical constituents that make it poisonous—are used in medications and even antidotes! Sometimes one poison acts as a countertoxin for the other.

In some cases, poisonous plants are also intoxicants. This power to change perception and to sway the flow of life and death is much like the power of the witch.

Some plants of the poison path are psychoactive. Some are magical and mysterious, encompassing long histories of ceremonial use and extensive mythology. Many are master plant spirits. They can act as familiars, helping us with our work. They are often teachers and allies, able to bring healing, often through the cycles of death and rebirth.

THE NIGHTSHADE FAMILY:
POWER PLANTS FOR MEDICINE AND MAGIC

Whether in Amazonian shamanism or European witchcraft, night-shades are valued for their power to facilitate spirit flight, visionary experiences, and communication with nonphysical beings. They are feared and respected for their power to move the life force and are of course connected to death and the spirit world.

What makes nightshades so important? Their family name, Solanaceae, gives a clue. As noted earlier, it originates with a Latin term meaning "to soothe." Nightshades can be analgesic, anticholinergic, anti-inflammatory, calming, deliriant, intoxicating, mydriatic, seda-tive, and soporific. These effects are dose dependent! For some night-shades, large doses may lead to coma or death. Other nightshades are only mildly toxic. And some of them give us everyday vegetables like tomatoes, potatoes, peppers, and eggplant.

Nightshades derive their medicinal, intoxicating, and psychoactive effects from their constituent alkaloids, such as atropine, hyoscyamine, and scopolamine. Some of these compounds are relaxing and sedating; they are known to relieve muscle pain and spasms, reduce pain, and decrease bodily secretions, among other things. For these reasons, they were important early anesthetics. Some are so powerful that they are poisonous even in small doses. The biochemistry of individual plants can be variable, meaning that one plant's alkaloid content can differ from that of another plant of the same species, so with the more toxic varieties, avoid ingestion. Topical application is safest (avoiding body orifices). They can be prepared as plasters, salves, liniments, and so on.

That said, magical uses for nightshades abound.

Magical Uses for Nightshades
- ✦ Binding, banishing, boundaries, blasting (a.k.a. hexing)
- ✦ Protection magic
- ✦ Cord cutting

✦ Love magic, influence, glamour
✦ Summoning spirits and necromancy
✦ Spirit flight, shamanic travel, witches' Sabbath
✦ Devil/Luciferian gnosis, illumination, and rebellion

Daniel Schulke describes nightshade effects as "gates of poison" from low to high dose. The first gate (smallest dose) offers exhilaration, stimulation, mental clarity, focus, and improved eyesight. Slightly higher doses become more aphrodisiac as inhibitions are lowered and muscles relax. The third gate is inebriation, when intoxication and perceptual changes begin to occur. This is also when some of the uncomfortable physical side effects like dry mouth and inability to urinate occur. Stupefacient, phantasmagorism, anesthetic, and fatal poison make up the last four gates on the path downward, and these last stages often seem to blur together. The visionary dosages can be precariously close to toxic dosages, and spirit flight and visitation occur during the deep soporific sleep state that can be achieved at median doses.

Gnosis may wait behind every gate, but the doors may also slam shut—proffering naught but agony and chastisement.
DANIEL SCHULKE, *VENEFICIUM*

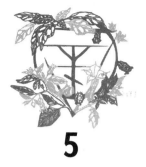

5

Botanical Allies

A Compendium of Plants for the Poison Path

*T*his chapter offers a compilation of some of my favorite baneful plant allies to work with. Not all of them are poisonous. Not all of them are psychoactive. Not all of them are harmful or adversarial or thorny. Some are even well known as beneficial medicinal herbs offering support, synergy, or balance. Yet all of the plants profiled here exhibit some quality of otherness. They have earned their place in the poison garden through their embrace of strangeness, potency, or resistance to being controlled. My intention is to show that this "banefulness" or "otherness" is a quality that courses through all of the natural world; it is not limited to plants that are poisonous.

Aconite/Monkshood/Wolfsbane
(*Aconitum* spp.)

One of the most potent botanical poisons, aconite has been known since antiquity for its deadly toxins. However, even this "Queen of Poison" as it was commonly known, has its medicinal uses. The prepared root is used in both Ayurvedic herbal medicine and traditional Chinese medicine to treat a variety of complaints including inflammation, pain, and paralysis.

Aconite was also an ingredient in Taoist elixirs of immortality as well as other popular drug preparations intended to increase longevity, promote ecstasy, and act as aphrodisiacs. These formulas often contained other potentially dangerous and psychoactive ingredients including: arsenic, psilocybe mushrooms, and digitalis. *Aconitum ferox* has also been employed for its entheogenic effects in India by small sects of practitioners devoted to Shiva, the deity associated with poison and intoxication. Even in this context the very real danger of death is not ignored, and the plant is approached with the utmost caution.

In both Chinese and Ayurvedic herbal medicine only the specially prepared roots are used in medicinal preparations, typically the variety *Aconitum carmichaelii*. The techniques of preparing the toxic rhizome, where the highest concentration of alkaloids are found, is done so to reduce the toxicity of the root before being used in medicinal applications. It is not recommended that fresh, homegrown roots be used in medicinal or magical formulations because the risk of poisoning is very real. Even handling the the fresh roots is dangerous because the toxic alkaloids can be absorbed through the skin. The root as well as the aerial parts of the plant lose the majority of their toxic compounds when dried. The dried and prepared rhizome can be purchased under the name *fu zi* through suppliers of herbs used in traditional Chinese medicine. When used in topical preparations aconite is valued for its ability to relieve pain associated with neuralgia and sciatica. However, it should only be used under the instruction of an experienced herbalist.

In Europe, aconite, also known as wolfsbane (*Aconitum lycoctonum*) and monkshood (*Aconitum napellus*), was widely known due to its toxicity. The plant caused quite a stir among the aristocracy from the time of the Roman Empire all the way into the Italian Renaissance. It was known for its use as a means of murder and assassination, and much effort went in to trying to find antidotes and prophylactics for its poison. The famous sixteenth-century *Poison Trials* of Pope Clement VII used aconite to test the efficacy of antidotes on condemned criminals. Not as much attention was paid to the action of the poison as it was to the efficacy of the antidote, but at the time the nature of poison was still not completely understood. The interest in poisons and their antidotes was a topic of interest throughout the Middle Ages, and inspired many to test their own antidotes on both human and animal subjects (Rankin, 2021).

Aconite was also one of the more commonly cited ingredients in the medieval witches' flying ointment formulas, when ideas of poison and diabolical witchcraft begin to coalesce in the years following the Black Death. While wolfsbane sounds like an ingredient that witches would be fond of there is some scientific basis for its inclusion in these recipes. With its pain-relieving properties and effects on the nervous system, it is not out of the question that this plant would have facilitated some kind of entheogenic effect, even a sensation of flight when applied with plants from the nightshade family, often found alongside it in the medieval flying ointment recipes.

Working with Aconite

This poisonous plant is unsurprisingly associated with the underworld and its associated spirits, including the goddess Hekate. It is an important plant ally in the witches' pharmacopoeia, and was said to have been used by the sorceress Medea to poison Theseus. There are safe ways of working with this plant ally and tapping into its magic and wisdom. Flower essences are one of the safest ways to connect with the energy of poison plant allies through ingestion; however it is especially important for this plant, that the flower essence be diluted.

Thankfully aconite or monkhood as it is commonly known has been cultivated and tended by monks in their monastery gardens, and you can often find it growing in churchyards. Especially those who employ gardeners with a nostalgia for traditional apothecary gardens. These are great places to connect with the living plant in meditation, which lend to its proficiency as an ally of introspection and solitude.

The flowers of the plant, once dried, are relatively safe to work with and can be carried as charms, incorporated into charm bags and talismanic jewelry. Monkshood was believed to confer invisibility to its holder, and can act as an energetic invisibility cloak when you need to move about undetected. It is especially effective when carried as a charm for protection during nocturnal rituals when discretion is needed.

Flowers and small amounts of dried plant material can also be added to anointing oils. These can be reserved for ritual objects or used to anoint the skin; however a sensitivity test is recommended to ensure there are no adverse reactions.

Black Hellebore (*Helleborus niger*)

Hellebore is another one of the classical witching herbs. It was used by the ancient Greeks as a cure for insanity and was associated with the mad frenzy of Dionysus and his maenads. (The insanity it was used to cure was often "women's hysteria.") An extract of hellebore was used in small doses as a purgative in early medicine to treat mental and emotional afflictions.

One of the most poisonous members of the buttercup family, hellebore was used as a murder weapon in the Middle Ages and thus had a malefic reputation. It was known for its use in ceremonial magic and necromancy.

Hellebore is connected to Lilith, Medusa, succubi, and other monstrous feminine figures. It can be used in charm bags to stop slander and gossip by its strangling effects. There is also some mention of the plant having the vampiric quality of being able to drain energy. I find hellebore to be very useful in daimonic workings.

☠ Caution ☠

Because it is extremely poisonous, hellebore should never be ingested.

❦

Brambles (*Rubus* spp.)

Growing in intricately woven thickets, brambles of all kinds grow at the edges of forests, fields, paths, and roadways around the world. They are hedge plants, occupying the liminal space of the boundary between cultivated and wild. They represent the threshold into the wilderness where all manner of spirits and beasts roam free. In many places, brambles are associated with the folkloric Devil and believed to be under his nefarious influence, and they have been used in many instances for healing and transference magic.

Folk customs say that it is ill advised to collect blackberries after a certain date in the fall, usually around the beginning of October. In Ireland, the reason for this is said to be that fairies or *pooka* have passed over them, rending them inedible. In Scotland and England, it is said that after Michaelmas (September 30), the Devil "casts his cloak" over them or "has been on them" (Watts 2007, 36). The precaution makes sense on a practical level, given that after the first frost any blackberries still present on bush are rendered tasteless and watery. Nonetheless, blackberry maintains its baneful reputation.

A bramble is obviously going to be a good ally for boundaries. We normally think of boundaries as keeping unwanted things out, but a bramble also asks us what are we giving away that we should be keeping for ourselves. It offers an extra layer of protection to help keep out unwanted influences when we are feeling vulnerable.

The bramble arch is traditionally seen as a gateway into the otherworld. It can help us achieve breakthroughs and cross thresholds on our own journey, offering defense and support.

Working with Brambles

Since blackberry and raspberry are both delicious edible berries, there are lots of potential ways to incorporate working with brambles. The leaves are known in traditional herbal medicine for their astringent properties, and they can be brewed into astringent teas and also washes for the skin. Blackberry canes can be cut and tied into bundles to dry, after which they can be burned to erect powerful protective/banishing boundaries. The plants in general help us strengthen our physical and energetic boundaries and hold on to what is ours.

Red raspberry leaf is historically a venerated uterine tonic that is still used today to help improve and protect the uterus during pregnancy.

✾

Darnel (*Lolium temulentum*)

Folk names: bearded darnel, delirium grass, temulentum (which refers to drunkenness), wheat's evil twin.

Darnel is a member of the grass family and resembles many of our grain crops. It likely originated in the Near East and once grew commonly throughout central Europe. There is evidence of an Egyptian variety dating back five thousand years, and it has also been found in Stone Age deposits throughout Europe.

Darnel's inebriating effects have been known since antiquity. Though it was often a "stowaway" grain, growing among cereal grains like oats and barley and contaminating their harvest, in some cases it was cultivated specifically for its psychoactive properties.

Darnel achieves its psychoactivity thanks to infection of its grains with fungi. Ergot is perhaps best known among fungi that infect grains and transmit psychoactive effects, but in the case of darnel the responsible agent is actually the parasitic rust fungus *Endoconidium temulentum* (Rätsch 2005).

The effects of darnel intoxication resemble those of tropane alkaloid toxicity and mycotoxins. They include pupil dilation, disturbances in perception, disturbances in coordination and movement, vomiting, headaches, sleepiness, and respiratory paralysis. These effects can last for days, though lethality is unlikely.

Darnel was known as "the plant of frenzy" in ancient Greece. It has connections to Demeter/Ceres and Persephone because it is a cereal grain, and it is thought to have been a used in various religious cults. It is sometimes listed as an ingredient in medieval flying ointment recipes. It has been used as a fermenting aid and was added to alcohol for its intoxicating effects.

Fungi-infected darnel grains were likely baked into many loaves of bread throughout the centuries, both intentionally and unintentionally, and one might surmise that the European peasantry was in a semi-constant hallucinogenic state (which would explain a lot). Modern agricultural techniques have practically eliminated darnel from other cereal crops.

Datura/Thorn Apple/Devil's Trumpet (*Datura* spp.)

The origin of datura is a matter of debate. The oldest species is thought to be *Datura metel*, which has been traced to India. It is likely that *Datura stramonium* and other varieties have origins in North America. In Mexico, *Datura stramonium* is considered a "younger sister" to *Datura innoxia*, and the two are used in much the same way. This may suggest the later arrival of *D. stramonium* in Mexico. While datura was written about in antiquity, albeit fearfully by Theophrastus, Dioscorides, and Pliny, it seems to have been unknown in the Middle Ages and early Renaissance, not being mentioned by any of the writers of the time. John Gerard wrote in 1597 that thorn apple was still a rare curiosity in England.

Datura is a powerful poison as well as a spiritual and physical medicine. It is one of the most important ceremonial power plants in North America and has traditions of use among Indigenous people across the continent. Datura is revered as a master plant spirit and great teacher, one that must be approached with respect. Some fates may seem worse than death, and three days of paranoid madness may come close as seen in many cases of datura poisoning. It is a plant of transition and transformation and a powerful catalyst for change; it is often used to facilitate rites of passage. A shapeshifter with many different masks, datura can be a reassuring grandmother spirit or a monster.

Working with this plant spirit can be very intense. In shadow work, it helps with fear-based anxiety, aggressive behaviors (also fear-based), paranoia, and nightmares, which can all result as symptoms of the intense work that is being done. When we choose to do shadow work, we are plunged into the darkest parts of ourselves and sometimes lash out in resistance. Datura helps with this, teaching us how to transmute toxic patterns, environmental influences, and toxic attachments.

Once used as an effective treatment for asthma, datura opens us up. Just as it opens our airways, our path of communication, it opens us up to receive information, energy, or insight in other ways. It can also be used in this way to break through blockages of stagnant energy.

Working with Datura

As is the case for most members of the nightshade family, we must use care when working with datura. Datura should not be taken internally except under the direction of a qualified practitioner. It can be applied topically for grounding, relaxation, and sedation and to draw out unwanted energies (it is usually applied to the feet or some other specific area for drawing out).

Datura has many spiritual applications, from cleansing and banishing to soul retrieval and working through ancestral trauma. It teaches us to tap into our unconscious through dreams and waking visions. It is a formidable ally; it brings fear to our demons and chases away harmful spirits and maleficia. However, because of its extreme potency, it is best to work with this plant gently.

Pharmacological Uses

Datura has analgesic, anticholinergic, anti-inflammatory, antispasmodic, deliriant, expectorant, hypnotic, mydriatic, and sedative effects.

It has ethnopharmacological uses wherever it is found around the world, treating conditions from skin eruptions to asthma. It is used topically and internally to relieve pain and to treat injuries related to muscle strain, nerve pain/damage, painful joints, and injuries where the skin is still intact.

Datura is also sometimes used to treat nervous and mental disorders. The flowers are traditionally used by the Chumash people of North America in a foot soak that helps with exhaustion and stress.

The entire plant contains powerful tropane alkaloids, and the alkaloid content can vary greatly across species and plant parts. The main alkaloids are hyoscyamine and scopolamine. In small doses, they act as sedatives, producing pleasing hallucinations and erotic dreams. In larger doses, they become psychoactive.

Datura flowers and seeds can have an alkaloid content of up to 0.6 percent. Dried leaves can have an alkaloid content of 0.1 to 0.6 percent. One gram of dried leaves is considered a therapeutically efficacious dose for smoking (Rätsch 2005, 210, 212). Four to five grams of dried datura leaves contains enough alkaloids to produce fatal results (Lindequist 1992, cited in Rätsch 2005).

Scopolamine from datura has been used as a truth serum because of its deliriant and hypnotic effects and frightening hallucinations.

Ceremonial Uses

Datura is one of the most important ceremonial plants on the planet. Its sedative, hypnotic, and visionary qualities lend themselves well to ritual use, but it can also cause aggression, excitability, and amnesia.

In Indigenous North American traditions, datura was often used combined with tobacco and used in smoking blends for rites of passage. Ceremonial vessels resembling datura pods have been found in archaeological sites across North America, and new research continues to bring to light the scale of the importance this plant held to Indigenous American cultures historically, as well as its widespread use.

In some traditions, thorn apple is used in shamanic rituals to travel to other worlds, the past, or even inside patients to retrieve healing. It is also used in divination rituals; its entheogenic effects allow the practitioner to communicate with spirits and deities and see into the other side.

Shiva, the Hindu god of ecstasy, intoxication, and poison, among other things, is associated with *Datura metel*. This species of datura is often smoked in blends with cannabis to connect with the deity in ecstatic trance. Datura flowers can frequently be seen on altars to Shiva.

Magical Associations

Thorn apple is a hexing herb associated with malefic witchcraft. It can be used in hexing and cursing but also can be raised in defense against the same. It is a great herb for protection magic because it combines the qualities of Saturn and Mars for a long-lasting and powerful protection spell.

In my opinion, *Datura stramonium* is the "witchiest" of the thorn apple species. It is the species most associated with medieval European witchcraft, and it has the wild, scrappy look of an untamed plant compared to ornamental varieties.

Datura is often described as a grandmother figure, but one that demands the respect of those who approach her. As a shapeshifter spirit, datura is often perceived differently by different people, and it can manifest in a variety of plant, animal, and humanoid forms.

The flowers of thorn apple are vespertine; they open at night, releasing their scent to attract nocturnal pollinators. The plant is connected to the moon, nocturnal magic, darkness, and the creatures of the night. Coyotes, moths, bats, and spiders all have an affinity with thorn apple.

As a divinatory herb, datura is a powerful ally. It helps us connect to our psychic senses and see into other realities. I describe the spirit of thorn apple as the "psychedelic shaman" of the nightshade family; it takes you on journeys to a different place than the other nightshades.

Datura can also help us connect to ancestors, access past lives, and process trauma. The flowers can be used as offerings, whether in the form of burning dried flowers or leaving fresh ones on the altar.

Jimsonweed

Thorn apple became known as jimsonweed or Jamestown weed based on the story of an entire group of British soldiers who, charged with pacifying a rebellion in colonial Virginia, incapacitated themselves by unwittingly consuming datura leaves. Their hysterical state allegedly lasted for a number of days.

Devil's Breath

Notes from Harold Hansen's *The Witch's Garden* quoting Von Aphelen in *General Natural History* (1767) on the use of thornapple seeds: "The whores administer to those who have the misfortune to fall into their hands half of five grammes of these seeds in order to profit from their madness." Thorn apple has had a long and continued history with sex work and can be a powerful protective and empowering ally for those who live in the demimonde.

Devil's breath is a powdered synthetic scopolamine used throughout the world not only to engender feelings of relaxation and happiness but also with malicious intent, such as rendering victims dopey or even unconscious in order to conduct robberies, kidnappings, and sexual assault. The powder is either slipped into a drink or blown in the face (this is where it gets the name *devil's breath*). The scopolamine in this synthetic form is very concentrated; less than a gram can kill a person.

Scopolamine is an alkaloid that is present in all of the plants within the Solanaceae family. However, it is most infamously known as the active alkaloid in the daturas. For example, scopolamine is one of the main active constituents in sacred datura (*Datura stramonium*), sometimes called devil's trumpet, which has white flowers that point up toward the heavens. Scopolamine is also found in a relative of the Solanaceae family, the *Brugmansia* genus, which is native to South and Central America. Brugmansia, sometimes called angel's trumpet, has large white flowers that point down from the heavens. It is of particular ceremonial use to South American shamans. For example,

Brugmansia suaveolens, one of the seven *Brugmansia* species, is used as an ingredient in sacred ayahuasca ceremonies.

Datura Ointment

- 1 ounce dried *Datura stramonium* leaves
- 30 ml apple cider vinegar
- 30 ml vodka
- 250 ml carrier oil
- 4 tablespoons carnauba wax

Begin by powdering the dried datura, putting it in a mason jar. Next, add the apple cider vinegar and vodka and mix thoroughly. In the time it takes you to read this, it will be time to add the oil. The vinegar and alcohol help extract the tropane alkaloids from the plant material so it is better infused into the oil.

Once you have added the oil, put the open jar in a slow cooker on medium-high heat. Fill the slow cooker with enough water to mostly submerge the jar. Let the oil infuse for 4 to 6 hours.

Remove the jar from the slow cooker and strain out the plant material. Pour the oil into the top of a double boiler and add the wax. Warm the oil until the wax melts. (If you want to do the entire process on the stove, rather than using a slow cooker, that is fine. The higher heat of the double boiler is necessary to get the wax melted.)

Now you have a large amount of standardized datura ointment to work with. You can pour it into smaller containers or keep it in a mason jar. The suggested use is 1 teaspoon applied to the underarms, the soles of the feet, the chest, or energy centers.

☠ Caution ☠

Begin with a small patch test to make sure you don't have an allergic reaction to any of the ingredients in the ointment.

---

৬ Datura Finger-Pricking

The dried pods of datura are covered in tiny spines, which become like sharp needles when dried. Handling these dried pods, I often accidentally prick my fingers. Noticing a strange tingling sensation travel up my arms, I am reminded of the consciousness-altering effects of urtication, or flagellation with stinging nettles (*Urtica dioica*) for its healing, detoxifying, and trance-inducing effects. The similar sensations arising from datura pods are due not to the spines alone but also to the tropane alkaloids, which enter the bloodstream with each prick. The amounts are very small, and they may have more of an energetic than actual biochemical effect. Some people may find the sensation irritating, and sometimes it sticks with you, followed by redness or itching.

Here, we are purposely pricking our fingers by handling a dry datura pod as we ask the datura spirit to share its power and wisdom with us. We might do this to get into a meditative state to connect with the plant spirit or other allies, or perhaps as part of a personal cleansing and grounding ritual. It can also work as a technique to draw the healing energy of the plant spirit into your hands to then apply to another person through hands-on healing techniques.

The easiest method is to sit in a comfortable position, hold a dry datura pod with the tips of your thumb and forefingers, and rotate it in different directions. You can close your eyes or meditate on the details of the pod. You can hold on to the pod the entire time or just until you feel you have made a connection. The idea isn't to stab yourself and draw blood; you will poke yourself just by handling the pod, without trying to, so there's no need to be too aggressive.

For healing purposes—to remove trauma, spirits of illness, and stagnant energy—hold the pod between your hands and with the lightest pressure roll the pod between them until you begin to feel tingling. Then put the pod down and use your hands for healing as you normally would, placing them on or over specific areas. A more direct method would be to combine this technique with also pricking the person getting the healing, taking the pod and *gently* tapping the palms and backs of their hands, arms, and legs, being careful not to break this skin. This breaks through stagnant energies, bringing blood and life force to the surface and moving it through the body. It also infuses the energy body/spirit with the spiritual medicine of the datura plant.

Deadly Nightshade (*Atropa belladonna*)

As its name suggests, deadly nightshade has been used for murder, assassination, and suicide for centuries. It has been used as an aphrodisiac, beautifier, and medicine for just as long. This plant embodies the dualistic nature of the witch, both healer and heretic. An herb of the shadow realms, deadly nightshade gives us the ability to see in the shadows, the gift of discernment by opening our "eyes." It is a powerful poison plant ally that offers deep introspection and has the ability to take the shape of our fears so we can face them. It reflects back our own shadows; its black berries are mirrors into our soul.

A femme fatale, fearsome warrior, and dread goddess, the spirit of deadly nightshade is a standard-bearer of feminine liberation and seeks to break the conceptions that patriarchy has instilled in us. Gender, sexuality, sovereignty, pain, trauma, power roles, and personal agency are all themes associated with this plant. As a plant ally, it can help us find the courage to stand fully in who we are, fangs and all.

Associated with Atropos, the Fate responsible for cutting the thread of life, deadly nightshade can be used ritually for cutting cords with unhealthy people and patterns, including toxic relationships and traumatic attachments. It is a master plant spirit that can assist in otherworld travel, specifically to chthonic realms, the witches' Sabbath, and the astral plane.

Belladonna, as deadly nightshade is also known, helps us explore the mystery of the connection between sex and death, both within ourselves and in the world around us. We can work with it in the form of a flower essence, anointing oil, or plant ally to heal trauma of a sexual nature, help reconcile submissive and dominant aspects within ourselves, and embrace sexuality in a healthy way.

Belladonna brings protection but also teaches that we are capable of protecting ourselves. It is associated with the Valkyries, battle frenzy, and goddesses of war. It has even been used in biochemical warfare to poison opposing armies.

Working with Deadly Nightshade

Deadly nightshade is potentially poisonous if ingested, but it can be worked with safely using topical formulas such as infused oils and salves. Growing the plant is an act of witchcraft in itself and can be powerfully transformative. Like the other plants in the nightshade family, deadly nightshade offers lot of potential for use in ritual and healing. Working with it slowly and gradually is the best way to understand its full power.

Devil's Backbone
(*Kalanchoe daigremontiana*)

+ A succulent native to Madagascar.
+ Cultivated as an ornamental; has established itself in the wild in Florida.
+ Proliferates voluminously; also known as "mother of thousands."
+ Connects with Lilith as the mother of legions of demons.
+ Aboveground roots can produce new shoots, seeds (16,000 per fruit), and plantlets that grow on the tips of its leaves.
+ Is toxic to cats and dogs.
+ Offers medicinal properties for oral health, preventing cancer, and treating ulcers.
+ Symbolizes resilience, rebirth, and continuation in the face of adversity.

Devil's Guts/Hellweed/Dodder
(*Cuscuta* spp.)

Dodder is a parasitic vining plant that, lacking leaves and chlorophyll, attaches itself to a host plant, through which it receives its nutrients. Dodder grows rapidly, creating tangling canopies of yellowish-orange threads. Its flowers are tiny and unremarkable. It can quickly overcome the host plant, making it more susceptible to other diseases. Once dodder attaches to a suitable host plant, its own root dies. It can attach to multiple host plants at once.

Like all members of the morning glory or bindweed family, dodder is a great ally for binding rituals. It can be gathered and used in witch bottles to trap spirits and other unwanted energies. It has the ability to convert whatever it absorbs into energy it can use. It can be incorporated into charms and protection talismans for absorbing and transmuting energy.

Dodder can also be dried and used to fill poppets for malefic workings to diminish the energy of a target and transfer it to another. This vampiric quality can be employed in a number of different ways in order to move and contain energy.

✿

Devil's Paintbrush (*Hieracium aurantiacum*)

This plant's brilliant yellow-orange blooms are like dandelions. Introduced from Europe, the plant proliferated quickly in North America. It is called devil's paintbrush because of its prolific growth, which covers fields and pastures in swathes of color while frustrating the cultivation efforts of farmers. It is a prime example of a plant that is attributed to the devil because it is invasive and an adversary of farmers. Devil's paintbrush is difficult to kill; cutting down one stalk will cause two more to grow from the rhizome. This fiery flower literally spreads like wildfire.

It can help us learn to master adversity, spreading our influence, thriving in the face of defeat. Hawkweed, according to Maud Grieve, has sudorific, expectorant, and tonic properties. It is bitter and contains flavonoids and pigments (Grieve 1931).

Pliny called the plant hawkweed because he believed that hawks ate it to improve their eyesight. We can turn to this solar plant to help illuminate what is unseen and get a bird's-eye view of a situation. It is a plant of illumination and expansion, and we can work with it in meditation and ritual to open the crown and third eye, bringing light to our entire energy system.

Devil's Walking Stick (*Aralia spinosa*)

✦ A member of the ginseng family native to eastern North America, with juicy black fruit and spiny stems; deer resistant.

✦ Often grows in disturbed areas.

✦ Grown in Victorian gardens as a "grotesque ornamental."

✦ Used by American Civil War doctors for antiseptic treatment of bacterial infections.

✦ Seeds of the berries are mildly toxic.

✦ Decoction of the bark is used to break fever through perspiration.

✦ Is emetic and purgative.

✦ Used in North American witchcraft as a blasting rod.

Elder (*Sambucus* spp.)

Elder is another baneful herb that has a dark and sinister reputation. It is believed to be bad luck, an ill omen, and home for spirits and witches. In European folklore, many taboos and superstitions surround elder, all aimed toward avoiding its maleficia and petitioning its spirits. In some traditions, elder is said to be a gateway to the otherworld. In northern Europe, elder (*hyll*) was considered a protector of the farmstead, preserving the harmony between married couples—an interesting contrast to its more sinister associations (Frisvold 2021, 248).

Seeking the aid of elder during shadow work is like seeking out the advice of a wise old sage. Elder will make you figure it out for yourself but ensure you stay on the right track. It can confer immunity, strength, and protection both spiritually and physically. It can be used supportively during times of major stress and upheaval to remain balanced and grounded.

Working with Elder

There are many easy-to-find formulas containing elder for general health and wellness. We can work with elderflower to connect with spirits of the upperworld for purification and to remove low-vibration energy. We can also work with elder to connect with spirits of the underworld for insight and grounding. Combine the two practices to balance celestial and chthonic energies. Find an elder tree growing in the wild and make regular offerings, tying pieces of cloth to its branches to transfer dis-ease.

The seeds, stems, leaves, and roots of the plant contain cyanogenic glycosides, which can be poisonous in large amounts, causing a buildup of cyanide in the body over time. Typically these compounds are destroyed when the herb is cooked or dried. The berries and flowers contain much smaller amounts and are commonly used in medicinal preparations, such as elderberry syrup and elderflower liquor.

Foxglove (*Digitalis* spp.)

Foxglove seems to be one of the more whimsical of the poisonous plants, being associated with fairies and the otherworld, but as we all know, fairies are not the innocent sprites we see in Victorian-era photos. Foxglove is a potent heart medicine both chemically and energetically. Its powerful effects on the heart make it both a life-saving medicine and deadly poison.

Foxglove is great for empaths. It helps with recovery from burnout and keeps it from happening again by teaching the heart how to control what it transmits and receives. When the heart is open, we attract abundance and flow in harmony with the world around us. Foxglove not only helps open and heal the heart but can also balance the flow of energy. It is one of my favorite plant allies to help with all matters of the heart, including heartbreak, emotional trauma, self-love, and more.

Working with Foxglove

Making a flower essence or plant essence with foxglove is a powerful way to connect with the plant spirit, and flower essences can be safely ingested and applied to skin. Apply foxglove flower essence to the chest to work with the heart center. Fresh flowers can also be placed in this area.

Foxglove is grown as an ornamental for its stunning spikes of bell-shaped flowers. Try growing it in your own garden; it's an effective way to connect with its spirit and work with its healing energies.

☠ Caution ☠

Foxglove contains deadly digitoxin and should not be ingested. Care should be taken when handling fresh plant material, to avoid potential irritation and transdermal absorption of potentially dangerous cardiac glycosides.

Foxy Foxglove:
Courage and Strength for Wounded Warriors

Plants spirits pop up in the most interesting and unexpected of ways. Foxglove is one that has surprised me recently in ways I won't ever forget!

I have always considered foxglove the jovial fairy spirit of the poison garden. It was never a plant ally I was called to work with on a deeper level, though I would use its flower essence for its heart-opening/healing effects. Looking back, I can see that foxglove has been with me all along. It was one of the first plants I found at my local garden center, and it followed me in the background during my travels through the United Kingdom.

Foxglove slipped into my world after a particularly intense plant *medicine ceremony and a dramatic inner shift. I had picked up a couple of flowering foxglove plants from a garden center. I was planning on giving them to one of my witchy plant friends and had them at my place for a few days. When I went to deliver them to my friend's house, one of the plants sent out a clear message that it needed to stay because I needed its support and it was going to see me through what was happening.*

In February 2023 my biological father died unexpectedly. We didn't have a great relationship, and his death affected me in ways that I was not expecting and opened the door for a lot of things that I never got the chance to have closure on to finally be laid to rest. In addition to that I had also begun the process of coming off of kratom, *to which I had accidentally become addicted to two years prior. Kratom or* Mitragyna speciosa *is a plant that has effects similar to opioid pain killers, something that I already had a predisposition of addiction to, but had been sober from for two years before trying kratom. I was also experiencing a lot of anger and feelings of abandonment because my sister that was living with me at the time was moving out of the country to Ecuador. To make a long story short, my heart had been ripped to shreds and I no longer had the help of the kratom, which had been numbing the pain. The plant medicine ceremony happened to coincide with all of these other things going on and I was in for a long period of integration and healing.*

I kept the foxglove plant next to my bed for its entire flowering process. I slept next to it every night, and it was there as a silent guardian for the integration process. Once the plant had finished flowering, I got ready to move and transplant it, and I was struck with the realization of just how much support it had provided. This is truly a plant of the wounded warrior and some of the most powerful energetic heart medicine I've ever experienced. Just being near the plant during this tumultuous time was grounding and reassuring, and I've never felt more empathy or support from a plant ally before. The plant had cared for me in just the same manner as I had watered and cared for it.

I did a second plant medicine ceremony with my sister, and I placed the foxglove next to the altar. I gave the plant various offerings and burned incense for it, and then I sat next to it, gently stroking its leaves. The soft, fuzzy sensation was both physically and energetically comforting, like having a teddy bear. For me, the experience was proof that even while still a deadly poison, the spirit of this plant is often friendly and willing to help us, especially during dark times.

After the ceremony, I transplanted the foxglove at a special spot in the cemetery I frequent, and I return to the place regularly. I will forever carry the spirit of this foxglove with me as a plant spirit ally, never forgetting its strength and support. It hearkens back to a memory of warriors standing together in battle and often dying for one another. After having this experience with the foxglove, I feel like I have a much better understanding for its spiritual medicine, and I will continue to explore its messages.

Ghost Pipe (*Monotropa uniflora*)

Other names: corpse plant, ghost flower, Indian pipe

Ghost pipe is one of the most interesting and magical plants of the temperate woodlands of North America, northern South America, and Asia. At first glance this waxy, pale-white forest dweller looks more like a fungi than a plant. Ghost pipe is not a fungi but has a close relationship with them. The plant has a single stem and bell-shaped flower from which it derives its name *monoflora* or single-flowered. Its ghostly pale color is attributed to the fact that the plant is non-photosynthetic and it derives its nutrients from the fungal networks of the forest floor.

Looking to ghost pipe's resemblance to the human brain and spinal column gives us insight into its medicinal uses through the *Doctrine of Signatures*, which gives us insight into a plant's medicinal and magical uses as well as its elemental and planetary associations based on the correspondence of the plant's physical attributes. This resemblance tells us that the plant works on the central nervous system, acting as a nervine. It is valued for its efficacy in treating disorders of the nervous system, including pain management, seizures, muscle spasms, and migraines, and relieves pain by acting as an adaptogen, allowing our bodies to respond differently thereby increasing our ability to withstand pain.

Ghost pipe was used by various Indigenous peoples of North America for its medicinal benefits. It occurs in deciduous woodlands across North America, but it is rare, so it is important that we use sustainable harvesting practices when collecting it. We can also work with ghost pipe as a plant spirit ally, and use indirect energetic methods of working with its healing properties including the creation of plant essences, wherein the plant does not actually need to be harvested. Ghost pipe makes a powerful plant essence for integration after healing.

✿

Henbane (*Hyoscyamus niger*)

Henbane had a reputation throughout the ancient world as an herb of magic. Its powers regarding prophecy and spirit communication were well known by the ancient Greeks and Germanic people, and it was especially valued by the Vikings, who used it in rituals. Its psychoactive properties led to its traditional use in an entheogenic context. By medieval times, it was among the flying herbs used by witches.

It has at times been named *insana* for its ability to cause madness and *hypnotikon* for its sleep-inducing and hypnotic effects. It was often used in a similar way to its less prolific cousin, mandrake, and was infused into wine, beer, and honey for its intoxicating effects, with both ritual and recreational purposes.

Henbane can help with all matters related to death and dying (including shamanic death), coming to terms with mortality, transition of the dying, the grieving process, and so on. It can relieve fear and anxiety related to death and dying, but it helps with nervousness in general and is available in homeopathic formulas for this. It is one of the safer nightshades to work with both internally and externally and can offer pain relief and sedation when needed (for example, helping one sleep or relax when nervous system is overloaded from emotions).

Henbane is traditionally associated with necromancy. It can help with all sorts of divination, especially scrying and spirit communication. As an ally for shadow work, henbane is friendly and comforting but unafraid to run headfirst into battle. It can help make shadow work less scary by reducing anxiety when we confront our fears, but it will also bring up those fears we have tried to bury.

Though most commonly known for its associations with death, henbane is also a celebratory herb, a plant of shamanic inebriation used in sacred brews for its psychoactive effects, and a versatile aphrodisiac. It can be infused into oil and used in erotic massage, offering pain-relieving, relaxing, and inebriating effects. Henbane seeds were once roasted in European bathhouses to promote a more erotic atmosphere with their inebriating smoke. The leaves and crushed seeds have been used for aphrodisiac purposes in northern Africa, often mixed with Spanish fly (cantharides) or cannabis.

The plant is also known for being used in more coercive forms of love magic, including mental manipulation and glamour magic.

☠ Caution ☠

Both henbane and mandrake contain potent tropane alkaloids, which can be toxic if handled improperly.

Working with Henbane

Henbane can be used in incense blends for divination, specifically involving the dead. It also is effective at charging divinatory tools and promoting an atmosphere conducive to scrying when burned. When burning henbane, add it slowly and sparingly to the charcoal to avoid overwhelming effects.

Henbane massage oils can be used for pain-relieving and aphrodisiac effects, and henbane tincture and its derived compounds are used internally for various gastrointestinal issues. It is important that these preparations be formulated and administered properly; however, precedent shows us that even nonherbalists can work with this plant with little danger. (That does *not* mean that it doesn't have uncomfortable side effects.)

Henbane can be a good option when situations call for potent spiritual medicines. When applied to the skin, inhaled as smoke, or taken in small doses over time, it can create needed chemical and energetic changes in instances where profound and immediate spiritual healing/ assistance is needed.

Parsley
(*Petroselinum crispum*)*

+ Worn in garlands in ancient Greece during games and banquets; thought to promote appetite.
+ Used as a funerary herb in the ancient world to decorate graves and place on bodies. That association with death lent parsley an ominous significance.
+ "To be in need of parsley" was to be on the point of death.
+ Difficult to grow from seed because "the Devil takes his tithe of it."
+ Considered bad luck to transplant parsley, which offends the spirit tending the plant beds.

*Note: See page 153 in my earlier book, *The Poison Path Herbal* (2021), for more information on parsley.

Poison Hemlock (*Conium maculatum*)

Hemlock is connected to Cain, the first farmer, an important figure in Sabbatic witchcraft. The purple splotches typically found on its stems are called the Mark of Cain. (This name also denoted the so-called witch's mark.) Hemlock is one of the classical witching herbs, and this was most evident in the British Isles.

Hemlock is a dangerous toxin that brings paralysis before death. It can be used ritually to paralyze a situation or to immobilize an enemy; for this purpose, one might sprinkle dried hemlock or hemlock seeds over an image or object before burying it or sealing it in a jar. It is also known for being able to destroy sex drive and can be used in spells to end a relationship or stop unwanted advances.

As a flower essence, hemlock can give us support when we feel paralyzed or depressed. It can help us create healthier boundaries and cut off that which feeds on our energy.

☠ Caution ☠

Great care should be taken when working with hemlock, and it should never be ingested. The fresh plant material is the most potent and should be handled only with gloves.

Rosary Pea (*Abrus precatorius*)

Other names: Buddhist rosary bead, crab's eyes, Indian bead, Indian licorice, jequirity bean, love bean, lucky bean, prayer bean, precatory bean, Seminole bead, weather plant

Many of the common names for this plant refer to its uses in jewelry, in spiritual practice, and as a standard of measurement. This fast-growing vining plant, a member of the Fabaceae family, is native to the tropical regions of Asia and South America. It has become invasive in the Florida pinelands, where it grows prolifically. Its large and deep roots are difficult to remove; however, the plant dies back every year.

The flowers grow in clusters of pink, purple, and white and the leaves are compound. A twining plant, rosary pea grows up trees, fence posts, and any other structure it can find. The seedpods start out green, resembling those of other members of the pea family. When the seeds are ripe, the pods turn brown and split open, revealing bright red and black seeds.

The seeds are full of the toxic protein abrin, which can be fatal if ingested. The outer coat of the seeds is tough and difficult to damage.

The seeds were used by Indigenous Americans in jewelry because of their bright color and as a form of measurement of weight because they are consistently the same size. In the Amazon rainforest, they are made into ceremonial necklaces. In India, Buddhist monks sometimes used the seeds to make *mala*, meditative rosaries. The red and black seeds are also used in the Yoruba traditional religion and related folk traditions to represent the orisha Eleguá, who is the gatekeeper to the spirit world.

Red and black are both colors of protection and power, and rosary pea seeds are believed to be extremely protective and empowering by the cultures that traditionally work with them. I like to think of the red side representing fiery, masculine Mars energy and the black side representing earthy, feminine Saturnian energy, both of which have different protective qualities. They are like miniature reversible candles, half red, half black, used to return unwanted influences and magical attack. These powerful little seeds can be incorporated into charms, amulets, and rituals for their powerful protective energy. They are great for countermagic and reversing spells. Interestingly, *crab's eyes* is one common name for them, and powdered crab shell is a powerful ingredient for reversal magic.

Abrus precatorius is also sometimes called weather plant because of its use in forecasting the weather. In 1887, Josef Nowack of Vienna claimed that the movements of the plant predicted detailed weather patterns before they happened. There are many plants whose flowers and leaves respond to changes in moisture and humidity levels, but *A. precatorius* was believed to predict even meteorological factors like wind speed, wind direction, and snow and fog. Data may or may not support Nowack's theory. However, the leaves of this plant do indeed make notable movements in advance of changes in the weather:

✦ Horizontal leaves indicates a transition in the weather.
✦ Leaves sloping upward indicate fair weather.
✦ Leaves sloping downward indicate precipitation.

This seemingly conscious movement of the plant in connection with the weather suggests some interesting occult properties and spiritual potential.

Sun Opener (*Heimia salicifolia*)

Also known by its Aztec name, *sinicuichi*, sun opener is native to Central America and the surrounding area. It is traditionally prepared as a fermented tea that is brewed in the sun and allowed to steep for twenty-four hours. This tea is said to aid trance and divination and especially connection with the ancestors and the divine. It has a special ability to help us look into the past to find ancestral wisdom. Interestingly, sun opener also has anticholinergic properties, which it shares with the tropane alkaloids found in nightshades. However, unlike the nightshades, *H. salicifolia* is not poisonous, which allows us to more safely explore the same states of consciousness induced by those nightshades. I would never recommend drinking a tea made from deadly nightshade, datura, or henbane, but sun opener is meant to be taken as a tea.

✿

Syrian Rue (*Peganum harmala*)*

Other names: haoma, harmel

Syrian rue thrives in desert climates and is difficult to cultivate. Its grayish-black triangular seeds are used in rituals for their entheogenic effects. Some believe that Syrian rue may be the plant Dioscorides referred to as *moly*. The plant shows up in pre-Zoroastrian Persia in the cult of Mithras. It was at one time called the "plant of Bes," who was an archaic apotropaic deity.

Harmel has been revered as an apotropaic, a spell breaker, and a magical and medicinal panacea since ancient times. It is said to be able to break the power of spells and also the enchantments of djinn and to avert all evil and evil spirits. The smoke would be inhaled to break the influence of a spell.

Syrian rue has also been used in shamanic divination to connect with "fairylike" nature spirits. The seeds have psychotropic effects, which are said to be sedative, narcotic, and mildly to moderately visual—similar to opium. Burning the dried seeds as incense is the most common method, though they were also traditionally roasted, powdered, and smoked. They were also taken as a snuff to help clear the mind and made into an infusion, called harmel wine, which had extra intoxicating effects.

Syrian rue has euphoric and rhapsodic effects and has been used as an aphrodisiac. It has also been described as oneirogenic, meaning it enhances dreaming. Its psychoactive effects are largely due to the presence of harmine and harmaline. These harmala alkaloids are primarily MAO (monoamine oxidase) inhibitors. MAO is an enzyme responsible for catalyzing the breakdown of certain neurotransmitters; MAO inhibitors slow this process. As a result, harmala alkaloids like harmine and harmaline can be used to prolong the effects of compounds like N,N-DMT, facilitating visionary experiences. Approximately three to

---

*Note: See page 184 in my earlier book, *The Poison Path Herbal*, for more information on Syrian rue.

four grams or one teaspoon of crushed Syrian rue seeds is effective for activating DMT in this way.

Caution: Due do its MAO-inhibiting effects, Syrian rue can have dangerous interactions with other plants and medications. It should not be taken in combination with other MAO inhibitors or selective serotonin reuptake inhibitors (SSRIs). People taking antidepressants, antipsychotics, antianxiety medication, sleeping medications, or blood pressure medications and people who are breastfeeding or pregnant should avoid Syrian rue.

❦

Tomato (*Solanum lycopersicum*)

+ Classified as a poisonous nightshade
+ Seeds brought to Europe from Central America by explorers; was a part of the Aztec diet as early as 700 CE.
+ Feared in Europe for being poisonous; before becoming one of our most popular foods. It was believed to be responsible for the death of aristocratic families because it was poisonous, but in actuality it was caused by the high lead content in the pewter dishware that these families were eating from. The acidity of the tomatoes absorbed the lead from the plates and caused death by lead poisoning. However, this mechanism of action was not understood until later, leading people to believe that the tomato was a dangerous poison. Now we put ketchup on everything!
+ Tomato worms were also believed to be poisonous and to impart their toxicity to the fruit.

❦

Trollberries/Baneberries (*Actaea* spp.)

A member of the Ranunculaceae family, baneberry, sometimes called bugbane or cimicifuga, is a woodland perennial and a close relative of toxic aconite. *A. spicata* is the species common in northern Europe, while in eastern North America it's *A. rubra* (red baneberry) and in northern North America it's *A. pachypoda* (white baneberry). Its red or white berries are the most toxic part of the plant. The roots are purgative, emetic, and irritant. Baneberry can cause dizziness, headache, rapid pulse, vomiting, diarrhea, gastroenteritis, and in rare cases convulsions, coma, and death.

Another important variety is black cohosh (*Actaea racemosa*), an important medicinal herb for Indigenous North Americans. It is traditionally used to ease menstrual cramps, premenstrual syndrome, and labor and is still used in herbal medicine today.

Baneberry, as its name implies, is known for its ability to cause quick and dramatic poisoning. According to *Poisonous Plants of Eastern North America*, by Randy Westbrooks and James Preacher, there existed no documentation on the toxicity of baneberry until the 1903 self-experiments of herbalist Alice E. Bacon. Bacon began her experiment by ingesting increasing amounts of berries, from one to three to six, and monitoring their effects. She noted gastrointestinal and cardiac effects with all of the dosages, and the final dose produced a state of confusion, dizziness, and hallucinations of shapes and hues of blue (Westbrooks and Preacher 1986, 55).

In the Norse tradition, baneberry was believed to be influenced by and possess the virtues of the most harmful *vaettir* (spirits) (Frisvold 2021, 249).

Wormwood (*Artemisia absinthum*)*

Turpia deformes gigunt Absinthia campi, Terraque de fructu, quam sit amara docet. Untilled barren ground the loathsome Wormwood yields,
And well 'tis known how, through its root, bitter become the fields.
OVID, *EPISTULAE EX PONTO. LIB. III. EP. VIII. 15*

---

*Note: See pages 86–88 of my earlier book, *The Poison Path Herbal*, for more information on wormwood.

- Known in the ancient world for its bitter properties; taken to counteract the effects of overindulging in food and alcohol.
- Acts as a vermifuge, repelling insects and critters; used in medieval inks to render manuscripts undesirable to infestations.
- Used to remove spiritual infestations and energetic parasites.
- According to Elizabethan herbalist John Gerard, wormwood is a good antidote for the poison of toadstools when taken with vinegar and can be taken with wine to counteract the poison of hemlock, the shrew mouse, and the sea dragon.
- Offerings to Hekate were said to be wreathed in wormwood garlands.

MUSHROOMS: MESSENGERS OF THE UNDERWORLD

Fungi are the great intermediaries of the natural world, delivering information about water levels, soil nutrients, and potential threats from tree to plant through belowground mycelial networks. Mycologist Paul Stamets compared the mycelial network to the internet in the way that it connects a multitude of different users.

Fungal networks are like the nervous system of a forest, sending messages for many different processes. Because of this, they have an intimate sympathy with our own nervous system, helping our bodies and minds improve the ways in which we send, receive, and process information.

Fungi offer powerful medicine. Medicinal mushrooms like chaga, cordyceps, and reishi are valued for their adaptogenic effects, which help the body's overall response to stress by strengthening the communication between body systems and creating a harmonistic synergy. Psychoactive mushrooms could be considered adaptogens for our mind and spirit, helping us process, integrate, and harmonize countless psycho-spiritual issues.

Mushrooms are creatures of the underworld, spending much of their existence underground only to pop up for a brief time here and there. They are strange and mysterious organisms, evoking fear and wonder in humankind.

✿

Devil's Snuffbox/Common Puffball (*Lycoperdon perlatum*)

You may recognize these mushrooms from the television series *The Witcher*; in one episode, a mage casts a spell and creates a bunch of puffballs that release a poisonous gas to quell the oncoming army. Puffballs don't release poisonous gas in real life, but their Latin name, *Lycoperdon*, means "wolf fart."

Common puffballs are not poisonous, and the young ones are often edible. However, correct identification is imperative. Puffballs can resemble young amanita mushrooms, some of which are toxic. The inside of puffballs is white and has a homogenous texture. The inside of amanita mushrooms shows an outline of the adult mushroom-to-be.

These puffballs are most common in North America and Europe, though they do appear in other parts of the world. Some Indigenous peoples of North America used the dry spores of puffballs as a dressing for wounds, taking advantage of both their antimicrobial properties and their ability to stop bleeding.

These fungi reproduce by releasing a puff cloud of spores when they are squeezed or moved. I used to find puffballs and play with them when I was a kid. They make great little guardian spirits when collected and placed around the outside of the home.

✿

Fly Agaric/Amanita (*Amanita muscaria*)

An entheogenic mushroom used ceremonially since ancient times, amanita is a powerful partner in shamanic journeying. It helps us remember our connection to the rest of the universe and imparts courage and personal power through transformation. The Koryak people of Siberia are perhaps best known for their shamanic use of this mushroom.

Like all mushrooms, amanita helps transmit information, and it can help us find insight in almost any area. In the Northern Tradition, amanita is associated with Odin and inspiration and insight he gained by hanging himself on the world tree.

In magic, fly agaric's spirit is seen as a trickster and messenger of the otherworld. Ravens and crows have similar qualities, and we can work with fly agaric to connect with these spirits and learn their lessons. We can also use this mushroom in ritual to connect with ancestors, past selves, and unconscious wisdom.

Amanita can be safely worked with as long as the species has been correctly identified. It can be put into smoking blends, ingested orally, or made into several other preparations. Microdosing amanita can have a wide variety of benefits.

Caution: Some other species of *Amanita* are extremely poisonous, but they have notable differences from the red-orange caps of *A. muscaria*. The two most deadly mushrooms in the genus are *Amanita phalloides* (death cap) and *Amanita bisporigera* (destroying angel).

Medicinal Applications

Amanita has anti-inflammatory, antispasmodic, aphrodisiac, muscarinic, neuroprotective, and sedative (or, conversely, stimulating) effects. They can vary depending on the dosage and alkaloid profile.

The mushroom is taken as a microdose to treat a number of mental and physical ailments, including neurological disorders, anxiety, insomnia, depression, and addiction. It is traditionally used in Siberia as a nervous system tonic and strengthener to treat exhaustion. It can be used topically to treat pain (especially nerve pain), sciatica, and rheumatism. It also can be used as an antivenom for snakebite.

Chemical Constituents

Amanita's main active constituents are ibotenic acid and muscimol, with trace amounts of muscarine as well as acetylcholine, muscazone, and muscaridine. The ibotenic acid is present in the fresh plant material but is largely converted to muscimol when the fungus is dried using heat. The remaining ibotenic acid can be further converted by decocting the dried mushrooms. Muscimol is regarded as the psychoactive constituent, though ibotenic acid has applications as well.

Ibotenic acid is responsible for the mushroom's stimulating qualities. It promotes attention, motivation, and focus. It is said that ancient Scandinavian berserkers used amanita to summon their battle rage; while some people debate that issue, to me that wild frenzy sounds like ibotenic acid. It is toxic at moderate doses and can cause the nausea and other uncomfortable effects associated with psychedelic mushrooms.

Muscimol is responsible for the mushroom's calming, euphoric, and pleasant effects. It affects the GABA receptors and the dopamine cycle. It can be toxic at high doses. Muscimol is a potent agonist of GABA type A (GABAA), the central nervous system's primary inhibitory neurotransmitter. It should not be combined with other GABA depressants, such as benzodiazepines and barbiturates, or with alcohol.

Amanita Mushroom Dual Extract

Amanita should be consumed only after it has been *completely* dried. The fresh mushrooms contain higher amounts of ibotenic acid, which can cause major stomach upset if consumed, so it is important that *Amanita muscaria* be completely dried before consuming or using in any formulas. This can be achieved by using a number of different methods; however pre-dried amanita mushrooms can also be purchased from reputable suppliers. As noted earlier, drying the mushrooms converts the ibotenic acid into muscimol, and muscimol is what we want.

The mushrooms should be cleaned before being dried by gently brushing with a mushroom brush or paper towel to remove any dirt or debris. The most traditional way of drying amanita mushrooms is air-drying, and this has been achieved in various ways throughout history. The easiest way to air-dry the fresh mushrooms is to place the fresh caps on a drying rack on top of a layer of paper towels or cardboard. The one drawback of air-drying is that it is a slow process and there is a higher chance that the mushrooms will go bad. Air-drying can best be achieved in a room that is warm and dry. If the humidity is too high the mushrooms will not dry properly. Additionally, you can put a fan on the mushrooms to help circulate the air and accelerate the drying process. It is also helpful to turn the mushrooms every so often to ensure that they are drying on all sides, and also to keep the mushrooms from touching each other and overlapping.

Using a food dehydrator is probably the easiest way to dry amanita mushroom caps, but it more expensive initially. The food dehydrator will ensure that the mushrooms dry thoroughly and evenly without going bad. The dehydrator can be adjusted to specific temperature settings and will ensure that there is no humidity.

The other option would be to dry the caps in the oven, but it is important to keep the temperature low and check the mushrooms frequently to make sure they are not overcooked. It is helpful to let the fresh mushrooms sit out for a couple of hours after harvesting so that they lose some of their moisture naturally. To dry in the oven, place an even layer of amanita mushrooms on a baking sheet lined with parchment paper. Place this in the oven, leaving the door cracked so that moisture can escape. Drying times will vary and it is important to ensure that all of the mushrooms are *completely* dry. They will have the consistency of a thick potato chip when completely dry. The oven temperature depends on a variety of factors, including the type of oven, the size of the mushrooms, and individual experience. In *Microdosing with Amanita Muscaria* (2022), author and amanita expert Baba Masha suggests a temperature of 109 degrees Fahrenheit to 131 degrees Fahrenheit, while other amanita enthusiasts suggest a temperature of 158 degrees

Fahrenheit to 170 degrees Fahrenheit. The World Health Organization notes that bateria are killed and prevented from multiplying at temperatures above 149 degrees Fahrenheit, while cannabis is typically decarbed in an oven at 225 degrees Fahrenheit to make the oil-soluble cannabinoids available. The latter is too high of a temperature for dehydrating mushrooms, since the goal is to get the moisture to evaporate, not to cook the mushroom in its juices. Some people will prefer a slow-dry at a low temp, which can take 4–12 hours. Others will prefer to work with a slightly higher temperature, keeping a closer eye on the progress of the mushrooms. I would suggest working at temperatures of 125–170 degrees Fahrenheit, and an absolute maximum temperature of 200 degrees Fahrenheit (with the door cracked). Most conventional ovens' lowest temperature setting is 170 degrees Fahrenheit, but some have a lower "hold warm" setting that can be used. Keeping the oven door cracked not only allows moisture to escape but also keeps the temperature from getting too high.

Like all fungi, which contain multiple compounds with different solubility, amanita must be double extracted (extracted in both water and alcohol) to get the full benefit of its medicine and convert the maximum amount of alkaloids. This is the technique that I use for my amanita extracts, which are made at a 1:10 ratio.

We'll use 50 grams of dried *Amanita muscaria*, with a desired end result of 500 ml of extract.

We'll begin by decocting the amanita twice in distilled or spring water. We call it a decoction because we are cooking it longer than we would a normal tea or infusion. When decocting, we boil the liquid until it is greatly reduced to make a more concentrated end result. In this case, with each decoction we will reduce the volume of water by half.

Start with 50 grams of amanita and 500 ml of water.

Add 20 ml of apple cider vinegar. (The acid pushes the extraction/conversion process further by lowering the pH.)

Bring to a boil, then reduce the heat and let simmer over medium-high heat until the liquid has reduced by half. This is the first decoction.

Add another 250 ml of water and simmer to reduce again. This is the second decoction.

Strain the mushrooms from the liquid, reserving both.

Set aside the water decoction. Place the boiled mushrooms in a pot.

Add 250 ml of vodka to the mushrooms in the pot. Heat over low heat until warm. (The alcohol evaporates quickly so we are just warming it up to help the process.)

Once the vodka and mushrooms are warm, transfer them to a mason jar. Add the water decoction. Let infuse for 24 hours. Then strain and bottle the extract.

The extract can be taken internally starting with a few drops at a time to connect with the spirit of amanita and get a feel for its energy and effects. It can be taken directly under the tongue or with a small amount of water. I usually start with 5 drops for a more energetic effect, and take 2–3 droppers for a more noticeable effect. The extract can also be applied topically for its pain-relieving properties. Observe how the extract tastes, how it feels in your mouth, and any sensations that arise in your body when sitting with it for the first time. The effects vary individually but may include the following.

Physical effects: sedation, bodily heaviness, stimulation, physical sensations, physical euphoria, muscle relaxation, perspiration, constricted pupils, increased salivation, pain relief

Visual and sensory effects: color enhancement, magnification, double vision, visual haze, external/internal hallucinations, synesthesia, disconnection, disassociation, cognitive euphoria, changes in libido, dream potentiation, empathy, increased sense of love and sociability, sense of unity and interconnection, existential self-realization, introspection

Amanita Plant Medicine Ceremony

I wanted to share this story because phytognosis is very personal and difficult to put into words without the context of the experience that

confers it. It must be experienced. The spiritual and symbolic associations we have, the ones we can tap into for strength, are often ours alone. I also wanted to share this story to give people an idea of what a full plant medicine ceremony looks like from the side of a participant, before, during, and after the ceremony. Every ceremony has uniquely personal elements, such as, here, the divinations, which bring more depth and synchronicity to the experience. What you will see here are my personal reflections.

Pre-ceremony Divination

Before any plant medicine ceremony I like to do divination. This could be runes, tarot, oracle cards, or a combination of different modalities. The meaning of the divination is not always immediately apparent during the ceremony, and usually has much more profound meaning afterward. However, it can indicate different energies, themes, or spirits that will be present in the ceremony. These can also be used after the fact to connect with what comes up in the ceremony. The following are three runes that were drawn prior to beginning this ceremony (see page 137).

"Anger is easier than sadness. Anger is an outward projection of inner sadness and pain. It's easier to lash out than to feel the pain. Every monster, every demon, is like a wounded animal needing love and compassion. Unconditional love is there, no matter what is on the receiving end."

The Ceremony Recap

Note: Names have been changed to protect the privacy of the other practitioners.

Something primal has awoken within me during this ceremony. I have fought many battles over a short time, which have led me to this point. As soon as I said I would do the ceremony, I felt tapped into its power. This was my first group ceremony. I had done plant medicine ceremonies and detoxes on my own, but this time it was different. I never thought in a million years I would be going through this again

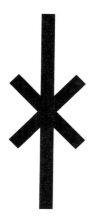 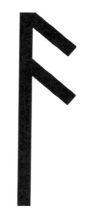 

Hagalaz: hail; a destructive force; confronting past patterns objectively; crisis; surrender; acceptance; radical change; Ragnarok

Ansuz: breath of Odin; transmission of intelligence; inspiration; answers; divine communion; *galdr* (spoken/sung spells); passing of breath along the ancestral line

Perthro: the Nornir; fate; a good omen; symbolic of divination cup; fellowship; also can represent psychological or emotional addictions; perception of *wyrd*

after my long journey of recovery, and I never thought that it would be a plant that brought me back to this place. Two years or so before this ceremony, I tried kratom for the first time. Kratom is a popular recreational drink served like iced tea all across the state of Florida, and is sold in dry-powdered form around the world. It comes from the leaves of the plant Mitragyna speciosa, *a member of the coffee family. It seemed harmless enough, and against my better judgment I would start drinking it every day until I needed it to function. Withdrawal sucks, and it makes you want to isolate, but I realize that we need to go through this process with the support of others.*

The ceremony began the week before with a typical dieta. *A* dieta *prepares you for the plant medicine ceremony in the days leading up to it and includes avoiding meat, sugar, unhealthy foods, alcohol, and sex. Some people will choose to fast, and abstain from other things including certain types of music to help physically, mentally, and spiritually prepare for the ceremony. This also helps to clean out the body so that the plant medicine can act more effectively. We were cleansed in smoke, fire, and water and by the plants of the earth. We took liquid tobacco for purging and opening our eyes and ears, clearing our sight. We painted each other's faces, something I had never before felt worthy of doing. We took part in the communal black drink, which began weaving our spirits and our songs into one. Honey mead, rose, amanita, and datura were powerful master plant spirits, along with Grandfather Tobacco. The smell of honey and mushrooms will forever bring me back to this primal ancestral place.*

Now, even long after, I feel so connected to the people who were there. All of the healers and other participants came together for this moment, after thousands of years, and I will never forget them. I feel changed in so many ways.

We fought for our lives. We cried, screamed, laughed, and healed together, each pushing through for the others.

Ragnarok Begins

After a week of balmy 70- to 80-degree weather, the temperature dropped. On the day of the ceremony, wind, rain, and thunder loomed in the sky above: a sign of Thor's presence and blessing. The storm was never too intense, but always present. We journeyed for the evening in a yurt. The ceremony was led by Patricia and Ryan, and we listened to familiar Norwegian folk music. War drums, throat singing, battle cries, and the runes being sung over and over—it took us to a different time and place. The music and its fluctuation between war music and beautiful singing had an intense influence on the experience, demonstrating the powerful dynamic expressed through the masculine and feminine forces that danced all night. We created energy, we gave birth, and we sent it out into the world. We moved the energy through us and around us in a powerful cacophony of ancestral song, our spirits and voices rising out from the peak of the roof into the night. Through the window in the roof of the yurt, the dark sky was tinted green all night.

Berserkir: *Amanita muscaria*

The amanita formula provided a powerful somatic experience, one that was very much in the body as well as the mind. Waves of ecstatic energy pulsed through me. A feeling of warmth and arousal rushed through my entire being, turning into a primal power that eventually became so overwhelming it came out in many ways. This happened in cycles throughout the night, alternating between everything from ecstatic emotional exhaustion to animalistic growling, with hissing, spitting, and gnashing of my teeth. This was, as described, an intense experience—one of the most powerful and profound of my life.

It was also a very animalistic experience for me, and I no doubt channeled the berserker strength and frenzy that amanita has been associated with. On one hand it aggravated my "demons," and on the other it gave me immense strength. I went there carrying things for so many people and became frustrated when my own monsters seemed to stand in my way. Ancestors living and dead, loved ones I've known in this life and in others—they were all there with me. They showed up for me, and they told me I had to fight for myself or I would never be able to help the people I was meant to. I've always tried to protect the people I love, often to my own detriment, and I have had to atone for that and pay the debts for the healing that I blocked through the abuse of plant allies and other substances as coping mechanisms. It is one thing to cope, but I crossed that line a long time ago.

Flying Venoms and Social Anxiety

Leading up to the ceremony, my biggest anxiety centered on the fact that this would be a group ceremony, in a new place with new people, and I wouldn't have my usual coping mechanisms available. I found myself waking up every night at 3 or 4 a.m. with intense anxiety.

I realize now how necessary the group experience was. About 30 minutes after I had taken the plant medicine, I felt the air within me shift and I let out a loud burpy growl. I didn't do any purging (vomit wise), and I was told Ryan purged for me at the beginning, but I was unaware of that. My purging seemed to be more related to the element of air, which makes sense because I smoke cigarettes and cannabis. I think I did a lot of purging with yawns, deep breaths, tears, growls, and snarls.

It felt as if there were two creatures fighting inside of me, a dire wolf and some sort of "alien biomechanical air-serpents." They were inside me, but also part of the fabric of reality in some weird way, like something out of The Matrix. *Not cute and not nice. I remember collapsing and someone or multiple people behind me pulling one of these air-serpent things out from the lower left side of my back (I'd been experiencing a lot of weird bubbling and swelling in that area in the previous few months, which had only recently started to subside prior to the ceremony).*

During a particulary intense part of the ceremony I stood there, seemingly held up by my very soul and I could feel Patricia come behind me places her hands on my back to move the energy. The literal fire coming from Patricia's hands was mind blowing. It felt just like hot coals, and I could feel it through the layers of my clothing. I remember flashing between hot and cold all night.

In addition to, or synonymous with, the weird snake things was another force inside me. Something that was watching the whole time, ready to strike. I have known this presence since I was a child. I felt dangerous and threatening and wanted to rip everything apart. I remember Patricia telling someone behind me to do something to "distract it over here." It felt like Ryan, Patricia, and the other healers were all behind me at that point, though I couldn't see them.

When I was at the peak of an aggressive outburst, Patricia came to me with a wind chime. I was entranced and hypnotized by it. It was so beautiful and so delicate, and I wanted to destroy it. As I looked at her face, to my left, her face paint changed from white to black, and I said, "You're trying to distract me." She moved to my right side, gazing into my eyes, just as entrancing as the wind chime, and said, "Oh no, on the contrary, I'm trying to help you."

Hanging on the World Tree

The questionnaire that we had to fill out prior to the ceremony had a variety of questions and one asked me which of three characters I was: Odin, Thor, or Loki. I picked Odin and I think that, by willingly doing so, I set myself up for a night of sacrifice on the world tree.

I remember Ryan's presence moving around the room, stalking like a wolf. I felt him come up behind me many times while the music was playing, but one time in particular I felt him working behind me. I could feel his masculine presence and support, and it gave me strength.

I remember seeing a lot of blood spatter on my hands, people's faces, and more. This seems to be something that is a common visual hallucination on Amanita muscaria, so it was interesting that I experienced this as well. The "wound washing" that I went through was also a very powerful process. An infusion of birch, a tree connected to healing, rebirth, and the Goddess was used to physically and energetically wash and heal our "wounds." It was like being nurtured after an intense battle. Being washed with the birch water was a wonderful experience and soothed the beast inside. I wanted to curl up in Patricia's arms. It brought me to tears. I could feel centuries of pain and trauma from warriors of the past and my ancestors. This nourished my soul and reached a part of me that hasn't felt this type of direct love since childhood (my mom stopped giving me baths a long time ago).

Valkyrie Rising and Blood-Eagle-ing

The Valkyrie spirit played an important role in my night. My wings were washed and made new and strong. I can still feel them. Previously, in the last ceremony I had done on the summer solstice, my sister mentioned that my wings looked like the wings of a hurt little bird, which was exactly how I felt at the time. Now they were magnificent, black-feathered gargoyle wings. I could literally feel my shoulder blades opening up and large wings expanding behind me. I felt Patricia reach into me and lift up

my body by my spine. She lifted me out of the battlefield and gave me a
new choice, among the three worlds. In many of the worlds' cosmologies
the universe is divided into three worlds: upper, middle, and lower. My
shoulders and back have since been sore, but they also feel more open
than they have in years. I feel taller.

One of the offerings I had brought for the altar was Atropa
belladonna, *or deadly nightshade, also known as walkerbeere or*
Valkyrie berry.

I had drawn a tarot card on the day of the ceremony, the Judgment
card, which depicts an angel with its wings spread (a Valkyrie) raising the
dead (warriors) from their graves (battlefield). When I drew the card,
I wasn't sure what it meant, but now the symbolic connection became
clear.

- ✦ *Judgment calls us to rise to a higher calling, indicating life-*
  changing decisions and experiences.
- ✦ *Judgments manifests when we reach a significant stage in our*
  journey.
- ✦ *Judgment helps us find comfort in sharing struggles within a*
  group. We can let them guide us and rise together.

The next experience reminded me of the "blood eagle" scene from
the show Vikings. *It literally felt like my back was opened up and my rib*
cage was flipped up in the back, exposing my lungs. Over the entire night
leading up to the ceremony, and even afterward, I had felt like I was
learning how to breathe again. This was some kind of atonement process
for overprotecting others, to my own and their detriment.

I had come into this ceremony carrying so many others—their
prayers, their love, their pain—and I realized to fight for myself is to
fight for them. I'll only be able to truly help the people I need to by
conquering my demons. I remember looking at my hands and seeing
them shift into the hands of many ancestors.

The entire night was like a birthing process, with so much feminine
energy that at times was uncomfortable and overwhelming. I felt like we

were all fighting for each other as well as ourselves; everyone's strength was shared. It was interesting to see the contrast between our individual experiences and our shared collective experience. I found myself feeling protective and guarding the door, remembering times in my childhood when doors could be dangerous and noises from other rooms meant something bad. The experience of group sleeping and collective safety brought a sense of ease; I was able to finally let my guard down at the end of the night.

This was an intense, warrior-culture experience. It was difficult and painful at times, but having gone through it, I feel stronger than ever: the berserker and the Valkyrie in one. I have been processing and reliving the experience over and over since the ceremony ended, and I see now: this is just the beginning of something entirely new.

HEALING HERBS ON THE POISON PATH

For obvious reasons, much of the discussion on the poison path is focused on poisonous plants. However, many healing and tonic herbs can be beneficial as part of this practice. As with all things, balance is key, and if we want to work with baneful herbs on a regular basis, we must balance that work with their healing counterparts. As we've noted throughout, poisonous plants do heal, but they heal differently, and their energy is strong. They create fast and dramatic changes, but they are too dangerous to be used long term. Tonic herbs can have just as dramatic an effect, but they work more slowly, building up over time.

Working with baneful plants in magical practice comes with its own set of obstacles and potential for disaster. Beyond the obvious risk of poisoning oneself, there are other ways that exposure to these forces can take their toll. It is important to understand the risks involved before working with any herb, whether medicinally or magically. If we understand the potential for side effects, interactions, and toxicity, we can take precautions to mitigate these factors and partner with other plant allies to minimize unwanted effects.

Poisonous and psychoactive plants can open us up to very primal and sometimes ambivalent forces. This is why it is always important to work with these plants in a ritual setting with a clear intention and clear boundaries. Disrespecting this boundary and working with these plants recreationally once you have entered into spiritual relationships with them can spell trouble.

The poison path is home to plants that bring shamanic (and sometimes real) death, herbs used in shadow work to awaken the hidden parts of ourselves, and plants that exist more in the land of the dead than in the land of the living. Our experiences with these plant allies are often very powerful, sometimes traumatic, and in the end cathartic if properly processed. If left in an unprocessed state, however, these experiences can lead to mental and spiritual disturbances.

Just as those who work with the dead must frequently practice proper cleansing and protection rituals, practitioners of the poison path should observe certain cleansing rituals and work with healing herbs to maintain their spiritual and physical health. Spending too much time in the land of the dead leaves its mark on a person, and the same goes for spending too much time in the poison garden.

When we immerse ourselves too deeply in the work of the poison path, the potential risks are manifold: temporary madness, mental disturbances, paranoia, melancholy, addiction (depending on the plant), and withdrawal from regular life. While working with baneful plants opens us up spiritually and psychically, it can also leave us susceptible to psychic attack and energetic parasites. When we work with baneful herbs, we bring their energy into our immediate vicinity. This intersection between a living being and a plant of death (symbolic or otherwise) creates a doorway that allows us to access numinous forces and experiences.

We can balance some of the qualities of baneful herbs and their aftereffects by incorporating herbs that brighten the mind, lift the spirits, and soothe the soul. A nourishing tea made from healing and soothing herbs can be welcome relief after a long night with a baneful ally. Here are some healing herbs I like to use.

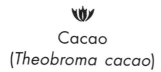

Cacao
(*Theobroma cacao*)

Cacao has been used by the Indigenous peoples of South and Central America for ceremonial purposes for centuries. It is considered a superfood and is rich in a number of important minerals including: magnesium, copper, calcium, iron, and sulphur, as well as being a source of antioxidants. It helps to support immune function, lower cholesterol and blood pressure, and supporting brain health. It increases blood flow to the brain and confers a sense of peace and euphoria. This heightened state helps with heart healing by causing a sense of safety and security for healing to take place. Cacao encourages the release of endorphins and dopamine as well as two key neurotransmitters: phenylethylamine (the love molecule) and anandamide (the bliss chemical. In combination these effects confer a sense of connection bringing us into our heart center and connecting us to those around us.

Through accessing this state of divine self-love we are able to let go of fear, anxiety, and trauma. Cacao helps to nourish the body, mind, and soul and makes a great supportive ally for intense periods of healing and integration. It is considered a food of the gods, and when we take part in cacao ceremonies, we connect with them. It is nourishing, nurturing, and healing and can help revive us after energetic burnout.

❀
Calamus/Sweet Flag
(*Acorus calamus*)

Calamus is a powerful herb in its own right. This reedy plant grows along bodies of water, and its fragrant root has been used in medicinal preparations to treat a wide range of symptoms, including neuralgia, asthma, bronchitis, hair loss, and more. It also stimulates the digestive system and strengthens the body.

Calamus root is used in traditional Chinese medicine to balance the energy systems. It is especially beneficial for the kidneys and liver, providing them with extra protection. This, combined with calamus's ability to bring clarity and fortitude to the mind, makes it a helpful partner for detoxing.

Vacha, as it is also known, is an important herb in Ayurvedic medicine and is used to treat a variety of conditions, from neurological disorders to respiratory issues and liver disorders. In hoodoo lore, calamus root is a root of mastery, used in formulas of compelling to gain mastery over people and situations. This use may derive from the manner in which Indigenous peoples of North America used it to bring stimulation, power, and strength to both the body and spirit.

❀
Lemon Balm (*Melissa officinalis*)

A tonic herb with versatile properties, lemon balm is held in high regard in plant alchemy, which connects it to the *prima materia*. The Primum Ens Melissa, a preparation of lemon balm, is one of the first and most important alchemical preparations. The genus name, *Melissa*, is Latin for "bees," which love lemon balm, and signifies the plant's connection to bees' transmutational power. Lemon balm is a relaxing tonic; it soothes the nerves and helps calm irritability and nervousness. It can be made into an infusion and drunk as a tea or added to smoking blends for its smooth and mellow effects. It helps soften the harshness of some of the more aggressive and fiery plant allies, like tobacco and datura.

Primum Ens Melissa

Lemon balm (*Melissa officinalis*) is one of the most important alchemical herbs. It can be taken as a tonic to vitalize the body and spirit, bringing healing on all levels. I prepared a lemon balm tincture and combined it with a 50:50 *Atropa belladonna* tincture, bringing the concentration of the *Atropa belladonna* tincture to 1:20. Lemon balm truly is a balm. It balances some of baneful belladonna's harsher qualities. By combining balm and bane, we achieve a powerful synergistic formula.

This sort of formula can be taken in microdoses in a ritual setting with a clear intention in mind. The dose is at your own discretion; I recommend starting with one to three drops taken in a small glass of water or under the tongue. (Or you can apply the dose topically, as you would a flying ointment.) If you begin to notice dryness in the throat, this is a sign that it is working. Don't take any more and see how you feel.

As an infusion or tincture, it can be taken twice a day to help with panic attacks, restlessness, and anxiety. It combines well with valerian and mints, like peppermint and spearmint.

Lemon balm is not just a physical medicine but also a spiritual one. It brings light and healing to the entire system. It has been used to drive away evil spirits and to promote a restful sleep without nightmares. It can be a welcome ally when we are processing cathartic experiences and going through intense emotional healing. It can soothe the heart after a romantic breakup or other emotional loss.

🌸

Rose (*Rosa* spp.)

Rose could be considered as much a symbol for the poison path as deadly nightshade is. It is also a common symbol of love and beauty, which belies a darker aspect protected by thorns that will rip and tear the flesh. Rose helps us uncover what is hidden within ourselves or protect ourselves behind a wall of thorns. Rose is powerful heart medicine; it heals, opens, and gently stimulates the heart center, facilitating self-love and opening us to the possibility of receiving the love of others. Rose helps the heart feel safe, secure, and nurtured, which is necessary for the integration of healing.

Rose is one of my favorite plants to work with medicinally and magically. It has both baneful and beneficent properties. The soft and fragrant flowers are soothing and calming, and they have a tonifying and astringent effect on the skin. Rose helps us strengthen our boundaries while keeping our heart open. Oftentimes we work with baneful herbs to process some kind of trauma or heartbreak. Rose is more than willing to stand by our side and offer us support during this time. It has nervine properties, calming anxiety and lifting mood. It also helps lift depression.

Working with rose after intense healing sessions and ritual work is a great way to both fortify and nurture the heart. We can bring the loving energy of this plant into our bodies by floating rose petals in a bath, using rose oil or hydrosol in our beauty regimen, or visiting a rose garden. We can also prepare rose as a tea, add it to a smoking blend, or make an infusion of it to wash our faces. Just the fragrance of rose has beneficial effects, though not everyone likes it.

Rose offers strong support and protection when we are too weak to stand up for ourselves, but it also shows us a gentle and nourishing side when needed. It is relaxing and mildly sedative, anti-inflammatory, and tonic for the heart.

Rose hips, the fruit of the rose bush, are rich in nutrients and disease-fighting antioxidants. They are supportive and restorative; like the rose itself, the hips bring strength, beauty, and protection.

Other members of the rose family, such as apple, blackthorn, and hawthorn, are also powerful plant allies for magical work.

NOURISHING AND GROUNDING HERBS

When we are working with potent herbs and entheogenic states of consciousness, it is important to keep our bodies strong, nourished, and fit vessels for plant spirit medicine. Maintaining a healthy diet and observing a dieta (a prescribed diet) before partaking in any major plant spirit medicine encourages a more effective and less uncomfortable experience. Fortifying the body and mind can also be achieved by working with certain healing herbs as part of your regular wellness plan.

Nourishing herbs are high in nutrients, minerals, and enzymes. They feed the body on a cellular level, giving it the strength it needs. Cleavers, dandelion, nettles, oat straw, and red raspberry leaf are all great options. They also gently cleanse and detoxify the body. You can take them daily as an infusion; let the infusion steep overnight to make it extra potent and to extract all of the minerals.

When our bodies are properly nourished, we feel better, have more energy, and can fight off illness and infection better. This also applies spiritually. When the body is strong, the spirit is strong and not as susceptible to outside influence. By feeding, nourishing, and caring for our bodies, we ground ourselves in them, become more aware of ourselves.

Poisonous plants awaken and open us to energies and spiritual forces that are primal and sometimes dangerous. Balance is key, as it is in all things. Incorporating a regimen of beneficent plant allies for health and wellness makes our relationship with other plant allies work more effectively. It also puts us into communication with our bodies, which is important for any kind of healing and spiritual practice.

Remember, *poisonous* doesn't always mean "deadly," and our baneful allies are willing to teach us many things. We must strive to understand each plant ally as an individual and apply it in ways that are safe and effective, in combination with other herbs that enhance the desired effects and reduce potential negative side effects.

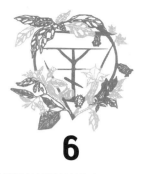

6

Formulary and Ritual Practicum

Building a Poison Path Practice

*T*here are many ways in which we come to understand the plants of the poison path, their spirits, and their action on human consciousness. In this chapter, we'll look at some of the ways we may work with these plants and come to understand them through formulas and rituals. Many practitioners utilize a combination of the formulas and rituals described here, and certainly no practitioner of the poison path is limited to them. This is my attempt to describe just a few of the more common ones and how they relate to the poison path.

TYPES OF PRACTITIONERS

The poison path is like a lightning bolt, forking into many-fingered branches. Though those who follow the path encompass all the diversity of humankind, certain characters or types of practitioners have emerged. These are not actual titles or categories; I have no desire to create labels or containers for any person or plant, and I don't think the spirits would allow it. It is simply informative to examine the ways in which practitioners have joined the path in order to fully appreciate the width and breadth of its reach.

The Entheogenic Witch

During the Middle Ages, many baneful plants gained a reputation for being associated with or even tended by the Devil. Their hallucinogenic and poisonous properties gave rise to their sinister reputation and connection to witchcraft. These were plants used in hexing, calling up the dead, and love magic. Their lore grew over time, and plants such as the mandrake became prized for their magical ability to find treasure or provide the bearer with familiar spirits.

Many practitioners of traditional witchcraft come to find the poison path because of their familiarity with these plants. These individuals who are well versed in working with both hands, understanding the connection between healing and harming, and working with forces both dark and light, find the allure of these plants enticing. The entheogenic witch uses these plants in spell craft, and the plants, themselves commonly associated with malefic magic, are all too willing to help in these endeavors. The witches' Sabbath is a central theme in the practice of traditional witchcraft, and the traditional witches' flying ointment (which we'll discuss later in this chapter) plays a pivotal role in helping the witch get there. Many witches come to study a variety of baneful plants for their uses in such ointments as well as ritual trance, spirit flight, and astral projection.

The Psychedelic Witch or Psychonaut

These are the travelers and shapeshifters, those who are well versed in achieving altered states of consciousness. Much of their devotional work and ritual is performed via some type of altered state achieved by using a variety of botanical preparations. This does not mean that these individuals are always high or that they need to be under the influence to work their magic. Tools as simple as using rosemary for focus and memory or mugwort for prophetic dreaming is part of their repertoire. There are all manner of plants that alter our consciousness and still allow us to be in control and go to work the next day. However, these practitioners can be experienced "trippers" and for important rituals may employ more powerful entheogenic allies such as cannabis, psilocybin mushrooms, or *Salvia divinorum*. They may combine these botanical allies with other techniques, such as fasting and ritual, to achieve the desired altered states. For further reading in this area, I highly recommend *Psychedelic Mystery Traditions* (2015) by Tom Hatsis.

The Shadow Worker and Death Walker

While these two categories are different in their desired outcome, they utilize baneful plants in a similar manner, taking advantage of the plants' powers over life and death to make the veil between the worlds thin, to loosen the spirit from the body, and to summon shades from the underworld.

These practitioners tend to focus on the plants that, through their myth and symbolism, are associated with the powers of life, death, and rebirth. They are also sacred to deities of the underworld and the dark side of nature. These plants can help us connect with these much maligned forces and also with the shadow within ourselves. They can teach us that there is much to learn from the darkness and death and that it is only our own fear that keeps us from mastering these primal forces. These plants can help us unlock deep insights within ourselves and, through communication with the spirit world, bring us new knowledge about life and death, light and shadow.

The Poisoner

The poisoner is part alchemist, part plant magician, and part toxicologist and has an in-depth understanding of the active components present within baneful plants and their effect on human physiology, specifically on an individual basis. They are the potion makers, extracting alkaloids from baneful herbs for the simple joy of their transmutation. They are the mad scientists, experimenting on themselves until they find the perfect dosage. They create tinctures and extracts that are potent enough to actually work, but safe enough that they may be used by a wide range of people. They make medicines for healing pain, helping with sleep, and soothing anxiety. These are the individuals resurrecting the wonders of these plants and making them available to the rest of us.

The Love Witch

Veneficium has links to Venus as the witch queen, presiding over all green knowledge. This is the other side to the poison path. Aphrodisiacs create just as powerful a reaction in human physiology and brain chemistry as poisons do. The love witch might infuse plants such as damiana and cubeb berries into wine or elixirs to make passions rise. They use psychoactive plants like mandrake and henbane for their amorous effect. These plants can just as easily stop the heart as well as engulf it with the fires of passion. The love witch exemplifies the double-edged sword of the goddess, who is both life and death, both love and lust. As we noted earlier, in ancient times, the words for love potion and poison were often one and the same.

APPLICATIONS FOR BANEFUL HERBS IN FORMULAS AND SPELL WORK

I am often asked by people how to incorporate baneful herbs into one's magical workings. The answer is that you can do so in much the same way as any other herbal ally. The following section provides inspiration for creating and experimenting with your own formulas and preparations. The plants of the poison path are inextricably connected to magical practice so their ritual applications are seemingly endless. Each plant has its own qualities, correspondences, and spiritual associations for more specific workings, but in general they are powerful allies that can add their potency to virtually any working. Let the plants speak to you, and don't be afraid to experiment while keeping common sense in mind.

Spell Ingredients

Baneful herbs can be dried, powdered, and incorporated into spell work just like any other herb.

✦ Add them to spell bottles, charm bags, or talismans.

✦ Sprinkle them to bring a Saturnian influence, obscure something from view, hide one's actions, or bind another's actions.

✦ Use them in spell work for spirit flight, shapeshifting, maleficia, and weather magic.

✦ Use them to enhance the power of other formulas.

Oils and Washes

By adding the baneful and otherworldly influence of these herbs to anointing oils, washes, or alcoholic spirits, we can incorporate them into our work in more ways.

✦ Use them to anoint the body, ritual tools, or effigies or to create magical space.

✦ Use them in dedication to specific deities or spirits.

✦ Produce oils or other infusions containing the plant's physical properties.

✦ Create energetic infusions or essences of the plants.

Flower Essences

As noted earlier, preparing baneful herbs as flower essences offers a safe way to work with them, even internally. We can use these flower essences for:

✦ Cathartic mental and emotional healing

✦ Processing trauma

✦ Overcoming anger and anxiety

✦ Healing and integrating the shadow

✦ Confronting fears

✦ Easing grief during periods of mourning

✦ Healing ancestral or past-life trauma

✦ Removing attachments

✦ Opening chakras and clearing blockages

Magical Inks

Baneful plants with dark-colored berries, like belladonna and black nightshade, can be made into inks. Or baneful plant material can be added to existing ink formulas to add their influence. We can use these inks for:

+ Writing petitions, symbols and sigils, and seals for summoning spirits
+ Writs of protection, banishing, and cursing
+ Staining and enlivening bones with plant spirits

Caution

With any liquid infusion or extract, care must be taken with these plants. Even topically applied ritual oils can have unwanted effects if not prepared properly. Be sure that you understand the properties of the plants you intend to use before preparing them as a liquid solution.

Spagyric Tinctures

Spagyric tincturing is a type of alchemical operation that creates an energetically powerful and spiritually alive end result. The word *spagyric* comes from the ancient Greek σπάω (*spáō*, "I draw, pull") and ἀγείρω (*ageírō*, "I assemble"), which essentially means to separate a substance into its basic parts and recombine them, *solve et coagula*. It was originally a technique of separating out the poisonous properties of a substance and drawing out and enhancing its medicinal efficacy. By doing this, we are enacting fundamental alchemical laws and processes, which transmute the plant substances we are working with into something different. We see the maxim "solve et coagula" on the arms of Eliphas Leví's Baphomet, illustrating this important concept.

Spagyric tinctures are effective on the physical, energetic, and ethereal levels. They are made at a therapeutic dose, meaning they have all the medicinal actions attributed to their phytochemistry. They are intended for entheogenic exploration, plant spirit gnosis, and spiritual/emotional healing. They are known for being more medicinally effective at smaller dosages, and they work synergistically because all the parts of the whole are maintained.

To prepare a spagyric tincture, alchemists work to create the *prima materia*, or first matter, by concentrating the salt, sulfur, and mercury of the plant material. These concepts represent physical processes and characteristics but also have spiritual correlations. Through the transmutation and exaltation of the formula, alchemists also transmute themselves.

The alcohol (menstruum) used to make the tincture represents mercury, the transmutational force. The sulfur comes from the volatile oils, alkaloids, and other components extracted from the marc (plant material). The *caput mortem* (dead head) of the extract is the plant material after it has been extracted; it represents the salt (the fixed quality).

A simplified version of the process proceeds as follows:

1. Prepare an alcohol extract of the plant material.
2. Separate the menstruum from the caput mortem.
3. Calcinate (char) the remaining plant material to ash. Typically the ash is calcinated until it is a whitish-gray color.
4. Add the ash (which is the salt) back to the mercury (alcohol) and sulfur (extracted constituents), which brings all the components back together after they have been transmuted.
5. Allow the mixture to tincture, then strain it. The remaining lump of material is known as the "vegetable stone," a kind of philosopher's stone of plant alchemy, which can be reserved and used for various alchemical and magical purposes.

Deadly nightshade (*Atropa belladonna*) is a poisonous plant. It is capable of causing death, but we seek to work with it to recover its medicinal applications, and also to work with this powerful plant on a spiritual level. I wanted to create this formula to offer something. By creating a spagyric tincture of deadly nightshade, observing the alchemical processes and utilizing lunar timing, we are able to bring out the spiritual, magical, and occult properties of the plant in a formula that is safe, effective, and easy to explore as far as dosing.

FLYING OINTMENTS

Flying ointments are becoming ubiquitous. Many practitioners today are growing their own plants and experimenting with their own flying ointment formulas, which is one of the most satisfying parts of the process! A lot of conversation centers on how to make these ointments, including questions of dosage and concentration, application, and the best carriers for absorption. There are many opinions out there, and many people offering techniques that have worked for them. The discussion below centers on my own personal findings, derived through research and experimentation over the years.

Uses of Flying Ointments

Flying ointments are entheogenic formulations. But these entheogens are wildly different from recreational drugs. They have a devotional aspect and are used during rites of passage to commune with the spirit world. These are not the giggly, feel-good highs of the recreational drug user. They are powerful psychic catalysts capable of unhinging the mind, enrapturing the soul, and freeing the spirit in a single night. Their use is not to be undertaken lightly. Proper understanding of how to work with these plants is developed over years of study and experimentation and is still not without risk. These plants have taken the lives of many an experienced witch and ethnopharmacologist.

Flying ointments have many applications in magic and witchcraft, including the following:

Traveling to the witches' Sabbath. "Traveling" to Sabbath is a visionary technique used by many witches, with and without the aid
of entheogenic ointments. The imagery of the Sabbat is of major
importance in traditional or folkloric witchcraft, and the source of
much of their lore. Entire traditions are built around the Sabbatic
mythos; this is called Sabbatic witchcraft.

Use as an initiatory tool. Just like in medieval witch lore, flying ointments can be used to initiate or dedicate ourselves to deities/spirits
associated with magic/witchcraft, such as Hekate, the Devil, the
horned gods, the queen of witches, the Fates, Medea, or Circe.

Connecting with plant spirit familiars. These entheogenic formulations can be used in meditation and journeying to help us connect
with plant spirits.

Honoring and connecting with the Mighty Dead. The Mighty Dead
denotes the long lineage of witch ancestors. Flying ointments have a
very long historical connection to the practice of witchcraft in general, and when we apply them, we are following in the footsteps of
those who went before us.

Preparing the body/spirit for chthonic journeying. We can use a flying ointment to anoint our bodies so that we can be accepted into
the realms of the dead, meet underworld-dwelling nature spirits,
and enter the presence of subterranean deities.

Invoking or summoning specific deities or spirits. Many of the herbs
used in flying ointments are known for their use in summoning
spirits. Combined with the entheogenic effects, these plant correspondences make the ointments a powerful invocatory tool.

Use as a tool of empowerment. Applying the ointment initiates a
change in consciousness and vibration, enveloping us in otherworldly power. We can apply a flying ointment to our hands before
a magical working or ritual to coat our fingers in the dark power of
their baneful ingredients.

Shapeshifting. Some older references mention entheogenic-type ointments in relation to shapeshifting. This magical technique can be

employed to facilitate healing, gather information, retrieve spiritual medicine, connect with other spirits, or enter realms where humans aren't welcome. Lycanthropy is an ancient practice that honors the most primal parts of ourselves. Warriors would use this as a technique to do better in battle, but also as a shamanic tool to channel aggression into something more constructive.

Applying Flying Ointments

When applying flying ointments, how much you apply and where you apply them has an effect on how they work.

You can use them to anoint your temples, your neck at the base of your skull, your chest, your underarms, and the soles of your feet. The only places you don't want to put them (nightshades and other poisonous plants) are sensitive areas, like around your mouth, nose, eyes, or genitals. The chemical constituents will absorb directly into the bloodstream. The more circulation the application site has, the better, and the larger the surface area you cover, the faster the ointment will absorb.

Another traditional technique is to first rub the site where you intend to apply the ointment vigorously with your hands. This encourages circulation, which leads to better absorption. When you apply the ointment, it helps to really rub it in. The heat and friction of repeated rubbing is going to help it absorb.

Most people say that it takes one to two hours for a flying ointment to take effect fully, but the timing varies from person to person. Sometimes you will notice effects almost immediately; other times you don't notice the effects until later or when you go to sleep.

Modern vs. Medieval Flying Ointments

The active components in flying ointments—the factors that cause the mind-altering effect—are the plant alkaloids. (There is a synergistic spiritual component here, but that is not the focus of our discussion.) The alkaloids occur naturally in a plant as secondary metabolites, meaning they aren't directly involved in the plant's metabolic processes.

However, alkaloids have a pronounced effect on human brain chemistry and physiology. Plants produce many different kinds of alkaloids with differing effects, but the alkaloids we are interested in are the tropane alkaloids.

Tropane alkaloids are characterized by the unique tropane ring in their chemical structure. They occur almost exclusively in plants of the Solanaceae family. The main tropane alkaloids are hyoscyamine, atropine, and scopolamine/hyoscine. These alkaloids have various physiological effects in humans and have been used medicinally for hundreds of years. Their effects on human brain chemistry and perception are due to their action as anticholinergics. Anticholinergics disrupt the neurotransmitter acetylcholine which regulates sleep, mood, and involuntary muscle function and this is the reason for the consciousness-altering effects of tropane alkaloids. You can read more extensively about anticholinergics, their chemistry, and their function in *The Poison Path Herbal*.

Medieval flying ointments were characterized by their soporific (sleep-inducing) properties. The visions and hallucinations that occurred happened during a drug-induced sleep or delirium. The ointments were also known for having an amnesiac effect and causing distortions in time. The accounts we have of these medieval formulations are dramatic, ascribing a sinister nature to the ointments, but one thing is sure: the individuals using these ointments were experiencing very real and obvious effects of tropane alkaloid toxicity.

So the question is, why are modern flying ointments so different? Why aren't witches across the country falling into a stupor after applying their ointments? A lot of it comes down to formulation, as well as the fear of using too much. However, a large part of it is due to the difference in the carriers we use today.

Modern herbal salve recipes use vegetable oils and waxes, which sit on the surface of the skin. This is why most herbal salves are meant for treating skin ailments and other superficial lesions. For better penetration to treat issues like pain, herbalists turn to a liniment, combining an alcohol-based tincture with an oil. The alcohol extracts the medicinal constituents from the plant and the oil acts as a carrier and helps keep the formula from drying the skin.

Tropane alkaloids don't extract as readily in vegetable oil as they do in other solvents. There are some exceptions and ways to overcome this issue, and alcohol is one of them. A liniment or some other alcohol intermediary combines the extractive power of alcohol with the versatility of oil.

The acidity and alkalinity of the environment the plant constituents are in also plays a role. Acidic solutions are better at extracting alkaloids into an aqueous solution such as water or alcohol, with the addition of apple cider vinegar, wine, or citric acid. This can be used as an intermediary method to help infuse the alkaloids into oil in which they are less soluble. Increasing the alkalinity of a solution helps to increase transdermal absorption of the alkaloids, which can be achieved by adding things like soot or ash to the oil. While oils do not technically have a pH they can act in ways that would be considered more acidic or more alkaline. Changing the pH of a formula in either direction can help with extraction. There are other vegetable-based options that are good for extraction because they are more alkali-like, such as coconut oil. By changing the pH, adding an acid or base to a solvent, we can create a chemical reaction that facilitates extraction, enhancing the extraction of the plant's alkaloids. Some vegetable oils, such as coconut oil, are more basic, while vegetable glycerin acts just like alcohol. Fatty acids contribute to an oil's acidity, which is why unprocessed or cold-processed vegetable oils and animal fats are better at extracting. For example, pork lard and unprocessed vegetable oils have a higher fatty acid content, which helps with extraction. Pork lard also has increased absorption. Because it is an animal product, it is more easily absorbed transdermally, which is one reason that medieval ointment recipes are more effective.

In the Middle Ages, the only options for an extractive carrier would have been olive oil and animal lard. These carriers would have been the basis for all medicinal herbal preparations. Animal lard, in particular, has much better absorption because of the similarity between human and animal DNA, permeability of lipids, and so on. Animal lard behaves more like an acidic substance because of the fatty acid content. I speculate that medieval herbalists would have used fresh plant material and "cooked" it into the lard, but I can't substantiate that, and I'm not sure whether cooking would eliminate the moisture found in fresh herbs and thus the threat of bacterial growth. Traditional herbal salves would have been kept at room temperature for up to a year.

We also often see soot mentioned in medieval flying ointment recipes. Soot or ash is used in fertilizer to raise the alkalinity of the soil and comes from carbonized hardwood. Adding soot to a formula would have raised its pH. A formula with a higher pH would be absorbed faster and better because the skin is naturally acidic; raising its pH opens the pores and promotes penetration of the product being applied. This same principle is used today in facial products.

So now we have optimally extracted ointments with a high pH, and we can see why they would be more effective than ointments made by other methods. Also, according to medieval accounts, the ointments were applied all over the body, not just in a few select spots, which would increase the absorption rate.

In conclusion, by taking a deeper look about what we know about phytochemistry and medieval flying ointments, we can see the slight changes that can be made to improve modern formulations. There is more than one way to get to an effective end result, and trying different techniques is an important part of the practice and understanding of the medicine these plants offer. This is not to say that vegan ointments made with vegetable products are ineffective, but that we must take additional steps to make those formulas work in the way we would want.

Notes on Formulation and Preparation

Flying ointments are easy to make in theory, and you can utilize any basic salve-making technique. Salves are made by infusing oil with dried plant material and then heating the oil along with beeswax to give it a thicker consistency. Vitamin E oil or rosemary essential oil can be added to help with preservation.

I use grapeseed oil because it already contains vitamin E and is practically scentless, but any vegetable oil will work. You can also take a more traditional route and use rendered pork or goose fat. I use one cup of oil per ounce of dried plant material.

When infusing baneful herbs into oil, it is important to use heat because the water-soluble alkaloids do not extract as readily into the oil as they do into water or alcohol. I use a double-boiler method to warm the oil: I combine the oil and dried herbs in a glass jar. Then I fill a slow cooker with a couple inches of water, place the jar in the water, and let it infuse in the warm water for four to six hours. After removing the jar from the slow cooker, I leave it to continue infusing in a warm, dark place for two to four weeks, taking advantage of both heat and time. Then I strain the oil, carefully pressing all the oil from the plant matter.

To convert the oil to ointment, I use one to two teaspoons of beeswax for every two tablespoons of infused oil. More beeswax will yield a thicker consistency, but I prefer a softer ointment with less wax. I store the ointment in one-ounce jars; each one contains the equivalent of 3.5 grams of plant material.

If I am making multiple doses, I place the jars on a baking sheet, add the beeswax to each one, and place the tray in the oven at low heat. Once the beeswax has melted, I add the infused oil and any essential oils, stirring the mixture to ensure it is thoroughly mixed, and then let them cool.

You might add essential oils to your ointment for aromatherapy or to enhance the action of the ointment. For example, you could add mugwort essential oil if you plan on using the ointment for divination or to enhance dreaming. You might add essential oil of clary sage, lavender, rosemary, or spikenard to enhance mental faculties, dream recall, and mental clarity; they can help with keeping focus and bringing information back from the spirit world.

Some practitioners add other ingredients to flying ointments for their sympathetic magic. Adding animal remains incorporates the power and guidance of the animal's spirit. Goose feathers or crow feathers can be burned and the ashes added to increase the power of transvection (soul flight). Powdered toad skin or snake sheds can be added to facilitate shapeshifting and for their connection to occult knowledge and cunning craft. (When adding animal remains of any sort, make sure they are finely powdered and use only minute amounts. These additives offer sympathetic energy, and larger amounts are not necessary.)

If you are adding soot, you might use the ashes of certain woods for their magical correspondences. I prefer using the calcined ashes of stems from the plants I am using. I use one teaspoon of ashes per cup of oil, adding it to the infused oil while it is still warm, before straining out the herbs. By using the ashes of the same plant you are infusing, you effectively create an energetically whole ointment, like a spagyric tincture.

৯ Flying Ointment Incantation

I wrote this incantation while making some of my flying ointments, which is when the plant spirits seem to be the most talkative. I get a lot of insights and ideas when I am brewing and blending witch's salves; I find myself connecting to that current of otherness. This incantation could be chanted during the creation of a flying ointment, specifically during the stirring process. I always stir my wax and other ingredients counterclockwise (against the sun) and was inspired by the resulting spiral of nightshade oil. It could also be used as a chant during a ritual to initiate trance for spirit flight or any other ritual using flying ointment.

> Swirling round the maelstrom go,
> Into the roots of the tree below.
> Fallen ones inside the Earth,
> Aid us now to bridge the firth.
> Bleeding snow and battle cry,
> Beating wings lift us high.
> By baneful balm and fates that weave,
> From the flesh our spirits cleave.

When we get to the heart of it, flying ointments are powerful botanical preparations that can be used in ritual and spiritual practice for profound insight and healing. When used in spell work or divination, flying ointments can be powerful allies. There is a lot to be discovered in trance work and spirit travel, and flying ointments are one of the methods we can employ to alter consciousness in a desirable way for these sorts of practices.

Medieval flying ointments originated in folk medicine but were chemically potent preparations that had psychoactive effects when used in a certain way. Today, we can employ what we know about medieval flying ointments and reverse-engineer them to adapt them to modern magical practice. Happy flying!

Beyond Flight

Flying ointments are part of the evolving mythos of the witch, and they hold many secrets and ways of working that go beyond trance work and soul flight. While the visionary states and experiences of flight are typical of the discussion regarding the medieval origins of the "witches' flying ointments," they are the backdrop to a deeper discussion of the implications of the beliefs and practices surrounding the premodern and modern use of these preparations and how we can draw from those beliefs and practices in new ways. Oftentimes when we open ourselves up to working outside the box, we open ourselves to receiving information from the plant spirits more freely.

This is not to say that magical ointments or "lifting balms" are exclusive to the witch. Psychoactive herbal salves, ointments, unguents, and ritual oils have been applied for myriad magical uses by different groups of people, for both benign and malefic purposes. They are used for not just soul flight but also astral projection, shapeshifting, dream magic, and dream incubation. They are even used for their aphrodisiac effects, such as inciting lust for use in sex magic and ecstatic trance.

Like all ritual implements, the witches' flying ointment is a vehicle for a specific type of energy. In this case, it is the energy of transgression and otherness that suffuses the nocturnal congregation of the witches' Sabbath. This is a liminal space between waking, dreaming, and death that we can connect with as a means of reaching greater numinous forces. While many of the traditional characteristics associated with the witches' Sabbath in the Middle Ages are influenced by Christian rhetoric, when we look back with a more informed gaze, we can cut away the overgrowth and reveal what is beneath. Not everyone will resonate with the imagery of the witches' Sabbath, and there are other cognates to this congregation of spirits, but for many of us, it is through embracing these taboos that we return to our more primal natures and connect with the numinous.

CONSIDERATIONS FOR SPIRIT FLIGHT AND OUT-OF-BODY WORK

There are many things to consider when embarking on any kind of spirit flight, especially with the added help of a flying ointment. As is the case for any plant-related ceremony, regardless of the intensity of the plants and fungi we're working with, not only are we opening ourselves to their spirits and allowing them within and around us, but we are also opening ourselves to other outside forces. In order for the spirit or part of the spirit to leave the body, it needs a road to follow. This tether, doorway, opening, or however it is described is a safeguard, but also a potential liability. While a flying ointment can be formulated to contain protective and supportive plants, it is helpful to take other steps to ease the transitions before, during, and after. The following considerations are not meant to inspire fear in this work but to provide additional layers of awareness for our ritual, beyond slapping an ointment on our skin.

Creating a Protective Boundary

By acting proactively and protecting the body, we are able to anchor ourselves to this world, where we aim to return upon completion of our journey. There are numerous techniques for creating a protective boundary or aura around the body. This symbolic and energetic boundary ensures that no unwanted influences attempt to disturb the body while the spirit is in flight.

Creating a container by demarcating a boundary, casting a circle, or laying a compass are all helpful ways to protect and ward the space. This could be as simple as drawing a circle on the floor or creating a circle of candles around ourselves. Ashes, soot, charcoal, black salt, and black chalk are my preferred substances for marking this sort of boundary. I use them interchangeably to create a protective container from not only outside forces but also inside forces, because we become portals when we do this work. In addition, covering other portals, like mirrors, is helpful to ensure there is no confusion for us and no extra points of entry for any other spirits.

Calling On Spirits and Allies

We can call on plant allies, familiar spirits, and deities for protection in both worlds as we travel. Goose, rabbit (hare), crow, owl, raven, toad, bat, horse (night-mare), raccoon, and possum are all powerful animal spirits to call upon. I personally like to work with the Valkyries, as they are able to traverse all the realms and are fierce protectors.

Cleansing

Cleansing and anointing the body with fragrant waters or perfumes prepares not only the physical body but also the spiritual body for flight. When we employ such rituals, we are not only washing the physical body but cleansing and blessing our fetch or spirit double before it goes on its journey.

Washing the Body

Washing the body is an important preparatory step for any working involving spirit flight, altered consciousness, or shamanic travel, but it's also helpful during or after these workings.

Create a simple herbal infusion and pour it into a large basin of water. Use your hands, a cloth, or plant material to wash your body. Work in an outward and downward direction: begin with the head, neck, and shoulders and work your way down the limbs, torso, legs, and finally feet.

The following herbs are helpful for this sort of cleansing.

- ✦ Birch: goddess energy, protection, Mother Earth, Berchta/Perchta/Holda/Venus/Freya—the Wild Hunt. The birch is a tree of regeneration, and those familiar with it will know that birch trees love to grow after fire has burned down the surrounding brush.
- ✦ Mugwort: soothing lunar energy, feminine/goddess energy, general cleansing properties.
- ✦ Yarrow: warrior herb, protection, courage, seals holes and corrects imbalances, helps seal the aura without compromising permeability (so we don't get locked in or out of our bodies).

Smoke Cleansing

Suffumigation (smoke cleansing) can also be performed before and after rituals of flight, and it's a great practice to put in place on a regular basis regardless of what you are doing. It raises the vibration of the energetic body and the ambient energy of the room/container. It appeases spirits and helps remove any stagnant and unwanted energies before any kind of spirit flight is attempted.

Herbs that lend themselves well to smoke cleansing include the following.

- ✦ Juniper: powerful cleansing and protective properties, tree of the underworld/world tree.

✦ Mugwort: general cleansing, psychic enhancement (helps with this kind of work), lunar associations, helps create a veil around the body/spirit so that we can go unnoticed.

✦ Resins: All resins are protective and cleansing. As examples, we can look to copal, frankincense, and myrrh. Copal is pleasing and sweet to the spirits; it is great for filling in the space after cleansing. Frankincense is very solar; it raises the vibration and elevates mood and energy. Myrrh has lunar associations and is more earthy/chthonic; it has been used in funerary preparations for embalming and as an incense.

✦ Wormwood: fiery and protective, especially for purging unwanted energy and getting rid of/keeping away parasitic entities and astral pests; can be prepared as an infusion for baths to get rid of unwanted influences.

Protective Symbols

Nightshades and other psychoactive plants typically used in flying ointments are most often associated with the planetary rulership of Saturn. This gives them a protective property, which is great for breaking and creating boundaries. They share this quality with soot or ash, which, as noted, was typically an ingredient in medieval witches' flying ointment recipes. It can also be added to flying ointments to darken them so they can be used to draw protective symbols in preparation for a spirit flight.

One of the symbols I find myself using often for spirit flight is the rune *algiz*, which looks like a broomstick or a person with their arms stretched out. It also resembles and evokes the imagery of the Valkyries. *Algiz* is extremely protective; it not only calls in divine protection but allows us to tap into the transmission of spiritual energies. It also represents the witch's foot or Devil's trident, the crossroads where all deals are made and all journeys begin. Trace this rune on the palms of the hands or the shoulder blades or use it to mark the bounds of the circle.

In addition to marking the body with specific symbols, you can also

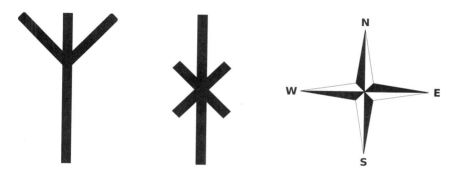

From left to right: *algiz*, *hagalaz*, and the traditional compass rose, demonstrating the crossroads and vertical directionality of spirit flight

use flying ointment, protective herbs, chalk, salt, or earth to demarcate the boundary of the body within the circle. You can draw four crosses at the four directions for a similar effect.

Herbal balms can be used to anoint the body to protect vulnerable areas or energy centers or to draw protective symbols on the body. You can also apply these balms to the palms of the hands to confer protection to others and carry the protective power of these plants into the spirit world. Good options include the following:

✦ Calendula: solar herb, good for the skin, smooths and heals the aura, brings light

✦ Lady's mantle: healing tonic herb, patron herb of herbalists

✦ Poplar: tree of the underworld, sacred to Hekate, protects both the physical and spiritual bodies during flight; historically a common ingredient in flying ointments

✦ St. John's wort: solar herb, balances energies, brings light, historically a common ingredient in flying ointments

Other Preparatory Measures

Another important consideration is where you are going and what spirits you intend to encounter. Having a destination in mind is helpful, whether it is the witches' Sabbath, the realm of the dead, or the dreamworld. Of course, the journey isn't always about the destination, and sometimes we fly for the sake of flying and the many pleasures it brings. Identifying your purpose will help you determine what sort of preparatory measures you need as well as what sorts of tools, weapons, and/or offerings you will take with you.

There are infinite gates and obstacles to be surmounted when seeking something in the spirit world. Each gate has its own key and each dragon its own weakness. A staff, wand, broom, or riding pole laid next to the body is a common partner to the traveler. The drum and rattle help encourage the trance state, move the spirit, and dissipate any discordant energy.

A witches' ladder is a traditional occult object symbolizing both the steed and the tree to be traversed. It takes a variety of forms and can be made from various components. It is, in essence, a vertical or linear arrangement of a number of tied charms, usually thirteen. These could be charm bags, feathers, bones, hagstones, or any number of *materia magica*. They are tied along the length of a cord, which usually has some prominent object of significant weight hanging from the bottom end. My own ladder is thirteen black charm bags tied along a black cord, with a preserved carrion crow foot at the end and three crow feathers placed intermittently along the length of the line. I hang this over my body or the altar and use it as a focal point for flight. It represents the axis mundi and thirteen moons and serves as a ladder to either ascend or descend the world tree.

When we enter the liminal places, we have to remember that we are not the only spirits that occupy this space and use it as a point of contact to the rest of the multiverse. Just like bus stops, airports, and subway stations, these in-between spaces serve as a gathering place for all sorts of creatures, and the same is true of the otherworld. Not all the spirits we encounter are the ones we are looking to meet, and there are also many spiritual parasites that unconsciously attach to those traveling through these places. Regular cleansing goes a long way toward not only removing attachments but keeping them from attaching in the first place. It always helps to have support, and we can call upon patron deities, familiar spirits, and other gateway entities to secure our passage. Another helpful practice is gathering dirt from a crossroads to incorporate into the boundary of the circle or container or to create a literal crossroads in the ritual area. This further enhances the liminal nature of the circle, and creates a symbolic crossroads that acts as a doorway for spirit flight.

Techniques for Flight

Flight does not necessarily imply an upward direction, and there are many ways into and out of the world tree. It is about finding the ways that work best for you. We contain within ourselves the same depths as the night sky. As above, so below; as within, so without.

❧ Behind the Moon

Visualize a vast night sky holding a giant full moon. The sky encompasses your entire view. Feel yourself being drawn toward the moon, or, alternatively, feel the moon being drawn toward you. As the moon comes closer, hold its fullness in your gaze. While holding on to this image, use your willpower to also attempt to look behind the moon to the dark side. Trying to hold these two simultaneous perspectives in your mind's eye will feel contradictory; push into that strange feeling, whether or not you're actually able to see the dark side of the moon. It's the contradictory feeling of lifting and falling, moving and being held in place, that you are looking for. Continue to explore this sensation in your meditations and see where it takes you.

❧ Falling Down

Flight often comes disguised as the feeling of falling, and indeed, we must fall until we learn to fly. Lie on a flat surface and become aware of the sensation of the surface beneath you. It could be the floor, the ground, a bed . . . Become aware of the pull of gravity. Become aware of the sensation of the surface beneath you in contact with the various parts of your body. Feeling

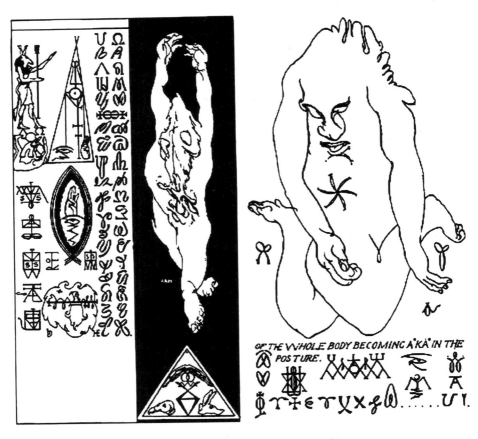

Death postures for trance work,
by Austin Osman Spare, from his book
The Book of Pleasure (1913; 1975)

the weight and consistency of this sensation, allow it to draw you down into the floor.

I typically practice this one lying face up in corpse pose, but you can also practice it face down. In addition to lying down, you can also employ the Sámi descent posture for underworld travel. In this posture, the traveler lies face down with their head turned to the left and their arms and legs outstretched. The right arm is extended slightly farther than the left arm, which remains drawn in closer to the body. The left knee is drawn up toward the left arm, while the right leg is only slightly bent. You wind up looking like you are scaling a cliff.

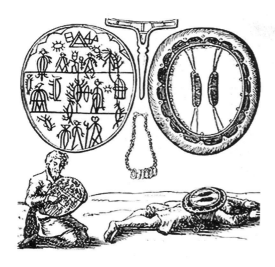

A Sámi shaman in trance,
as depicted in Jarving 2004

❧ The Hanged One

This technique can be employed for travel to not only the otherworld but various destinations. It draws on the imagery of the painting of the Hanged Man by Pamela Colman Smith as one of the major arcana in the Rider-Waite Tarot. When we look at the symbolism of this image, we see numerous connections to shamanic travel and the world tree.

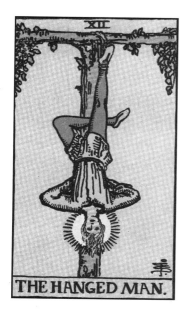

The Hanged Man, by
Pamela Colman Smith for
the Rider-Waite Tarot,
depicting a shamanic
trance posture

In this posture, the traveler lies on their back, facing up, with their right leg extended, the left leg bent, and the sole of the left foot placed near the right knee, creating a number 4 shape. Their hands are then placed behind the back at the base of the spine, one over the other. They may then also close their left eye or take it a step further and use something to cover the left eye completely.

Grounding

Spirit flight can be a disorienting experience so it is important to have some grounding practices in place when you return to normal consciousness. This helps to prevent the sense of still being out of one's body and helps to fully bring us back into the material realm. When it comes to spirit flight, much of the focus is placed on the plants and practices to help you achieve flight but there are also a number of allies and practices that help ease the landing as well.

+ Potato (*Solanum tuberosum*): grounding, protection, earth connection, and integrating intense spiritual experiences. In his book *Flower Essences from the Witch's Garden*, Nicholas Pearson goes into detail on the uses of potato as a flower essence for grounding. Whether energetically or as a food, potato grounds and nourishes us.
+ Salt baths: All salt has grounding and purifying properties, including sea salt, Himalayan salt, and Epsom salt. Any salt can be dissolved in a bath for its grounding properties.
+ Activated charcoal: Use like salt in a bath for its grounding properties. Activated charcoal can also be taken internally; mix a small amount into a glass of water and drink it. Activated charcoal is commonly sold as a dietary supplement.
+ Meat/protein, greasy or salty food, and CARBS! All of the things that we are typically told to avoid in our diet are also the things that can help bring us back into our body and ground us into the pleasures of the material world after traveling in spirit. Just

remember to take it slow; after coming off a long fast or dieta, eating an entire cheese pizza is not going to feel great. Trust me.

SITTING OUT WITH PLANT SPIRIT ALLIES AND LAND SPIRITS

Known as *utesitta* in Old Norse or *útiseta* in Icelandic, the custom of "sitting out"—going to mounds and other power places to make offerings and connect with land spirits—was common across northern Europe. A person would go to one of these power places alone, at night, and hold vigil until dawn, making offerings and speaking incantations over the course of the night in search of spirit visitations. *Utesitta* could be practiced at any place of power, including a crossroads, where it was associated with communing with the spirits of the dead (Frisvold 2021, 207).

Among the Germanic peoples, sitting out was associated with *seidr*, or prophetic sorcery achieved through the use of trance and shamanic ecstasy. Rooted in a connection with the spirits of the land, the *völva* (seeress) would work with the Nornir and other primal forces to bring about change and to prophesy (Frisvold 2021, 213). This was considered a feminine practice; it was considered dishonorable for men to practice sorcery in the warrior culture of Germanic peoples. *Seidr*, associated with the goddess Freya, was taught to Odin, but even he is ridiculed for the practice and called *ergi*, or unmanly. As Shani Oates explains in *The Hanged God*, "As an activity not focused upon war and warfare, Seidr was deemed too passive for manly engagement. So, despite the extreme power and respect recognized in female practitioners of Seidr, it bore the stigma of dishonor for a man to embody its secrets" (Oates 2022, 135). Today, it is with great pride that we break these misogynist constructs.

The concept of sitting out can be applied to working with plant spirit familiars, land spirits, and plant spirit medicine, offering powerful visionary and numinous experiences.

Plant Spirit Origins and Human Interaction

Plant spirits are our oldest ancestors and our most loyal allies. Plants are the original inhabitants of the Earth, and they carry with them a primordial wisdom. They provide us with medicine, nourishment, and shelter (look at the myriad ways in which we interact with plants in our day-to-day lives without even realizing it). While humankind has not always respected this relationship with the plant kingdom, exploiting its resources, plants continue to give themselves to humanity. Over the course of millennia, our relationship with the plants around us has directly influenced the evolution of humankind. Ethnobotanical research looks at how different cultures have utilized plants in spirituality and medicine throughout history. This ancient knowledge has almost been lost to time and the rise of modern medicine, but it is being recovered by those who answer the call of nature's wisdom.

The spiritual connection between humans and plants is evident in mythology. The origin myths of many plants tell of them springing up from the blood of heroes and deities. Some plants have a divine or infernal origin in mythology. And we see many cases of humans being transformed into plants and trees.

CONNECTING WITH PLANT SPIRIT FAMILIARS

Witches are known for partnering with all sorts of spirits to aid in their magical pursuits: plant, animal, and otherwise. These interactions, when continued on a regular basis, become a familiar relationship. Spirit familiars are trusted allies, teachers, and protectors that we can have deep and meaningful relationships with. They offer additional power and knowledge in exchange for energy, offerings, and the opportunity to cocreate with humans. This is a mutually beneficial relationship that facilitates the spiritual growth of both parties.

Spirit familiars take different forms and have different meanings in different cultures. They even appear differently to different practitioners. In traditional witchcraft lore, they would often take the form of an animal, though they can also take on the shape of a humanoid shadowy figure, the likeness of the witch, or any other anthropomorphic form.

Just like any other spirit familiar, plant spirit familiars act as teachers and guides. They manifest in different ways to different people, helping us learn and grow while elevating our craft. A witch's partnership with a plant spirit familiar generally lasts a lifetime.

Ways to Court a Plant Spirit Familiar

• Make regular contact with the plant spirit through meditation, ritual, and offerings.
• Offer to make a pact, coming to an agreement with the plant spirit to work in partnership.
• Prepare a physical vessel for the plant spirit to contain its physical, energetic, and spiritual bodies.
• Fashion the roots and stems of the plant into an effigy to house the plant spirit. The living plant is the most natural vessel for the plant spirit.
• Use liquid vessels, such as tinctures or infusions, to transfer the plant's spirit to other objects.
• Create glyphs and sigils for the plant, using ritual ink empowered by the actual plant material to draw them.

The Witch's Garden

More and more people are beginning to cultivate their own witch's garden containing many of the plants discussed throughout this book. The otherworldly beauty of these plants is undeniable. Their dark greens, dusty reds, and deep purples are beautiful to behold. Few places are more magical than a witch's garden under the light of the full moon.

Night-blooming datura and moonflowers release their intoxicatingly sweet scent, making it a place perfect for nocturnal meditation and reverie. Those who grow a witch's garden come to understand these plants most intimately because they get to experience them throughout their life cycle. Starting a plant from seed and caring for it over its life cycle forges a strong bond. The spirits of these plants make willing familiars and have much to teach those who approach them without fear. I highly recommend beginning your own witch's garden if you are interested in learning more about these plants. The best way to learn about their personalities is from the plants themselves.

Plant Spirit Vessels

Many practitioners create a vessel that serves as a home for their plant spirit familiar. A plant spirit vessel acts as a container for the power and intelligence of a plant spirit familiar. When we harvest a plant for its magical properties, it loses some of its life force and its connection to the greater plant spirit because its connection to the living plant has been severed. A plant spirit vessel restores this connection and life force by providing a new container for the body of the plant, serving as a proxy to the living plant. We keep these vessels on the altar after we have ritually consecrated and enlivened them. They are vessels for the living plant spirit and play a pivotal role in the rituals of the green witch, adding their power to spell work, potentiating and activating formulas, and serving as oracular devices.

The spirit vessel is much more than a container; it is a manifestation point, a physical meeting space where the spirit can anchor itself and draw energy. The spirit vessel acts as a battery, growing in power and connection as we work with it on a regular basis. As the place where we regularly congress with this plant spirit, the vessel becomes more connected to us and to the spirit. It can be used as a focal point for meditation to gain insight from the plant spirit familiar in the same way we would meditate with the living plant. It becomes a way for us to maintain a dialogue with the plant spirit. Once we begin working with a plant spirit regularly, it will take us down many different avenues, introducing us to new spirits through its own mythos.

A plant spirit vessel has its own unique anatomy, and each part of that anatomy has its own application, which, together, make up the whole of its potential. There is the daemon of the plant that inhabits the vessel, which is its own separate entity offering its own interaction. Think of this as the sulfur or fire that gives the vessel life. Then there is the physical aspect, composed of the vessel and plant matter, that we employ as a ritual or divinatory tool. We can consider this the salt. The liquid is its own entity, a spagyric tincture combined with the vital force and consciousness of the plant spirit familiar. This is the mercury, the binding agent that connects the physical and spiritual aspects. These three aspects combined and ritually prepared create a spiritual tool with vast potential.

Creating a plant spirit vessel is a powerful bonding opportunity, establishing an energetic and spiritual connection between plant and practitioner. The process can be used to strengthen a connection to an existing plant spirit familiar or one that you are just beginning to work with. After creating the plant spirit vessel, you will have successfully worked with all parts of the plant in a physical and spiritual capacity. Throughout the entire process, you are channeling the genius of the plant spirit, acting as a living intermediary for the plant while it is in transition into its new vessel.

Some practitioners ingest the herb in some way while constructing the vessel. This could be done through any of the usual means that are safe and appropriate for the plant you are working with. Doing this will bring that plant's vibration into your energy field so that the two of you can work together to create this sacred artifact.

Salt: The Physical Vessel

The vessel can be as ornate or as simple as you desire. Amber or colored glass, clasp jars, or waterproof clay vessels are all options. Avoid metal lids (for the vessel and throughout the entire process of preparing one) so that the influence of the metal is not imparted into the liquid carrier. If you are going to use the vessel as a surface for scrying, a large mason jar or other jar with a smooth surface works best. Also keep in mind that colored glass is pretty and will protect the liquid from sunlight, but you also won't be able to see the plant material floating around in the jar. This is one of the reasons I leave all the pieces whole—I like to see their unique character floating in the liquid.

You can decorate and adorn the vessel according to your personal preference and communion with the plant spirit. You might use charms, plant spirit glyphs, binding runes, and other power symbols. You might also consider covering the vessel in a shroud when not in use.

Plant glyphs are symbolic representations of plant spirit power that can act as connection points to specific currents of energy in meditation and ritual. The glyphs are created in congress with the genius of each plant ally. You can use a basic sigil-making technique and the plant's common or scientific names to create a symbol. They are meant to be shared and used so that they grow in power. You can use mine or create your own.

The plant spirit vessel is in essence a more complex version of

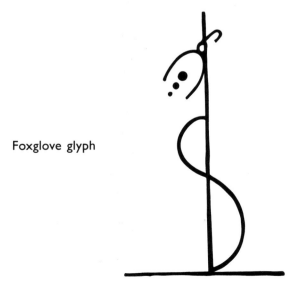

Foxglove glyph

the plant spirit glyph, and the two can be combined to enhance their power. Use the plant spirit glyph to adorn the vessel or incorporate it into the ritual of construction. The glyph can serve as your own symbol for identifying the contents of the vessel; remember, there is power in hidden things.

You can ritually activate and empower the vessel you create by placing it over planetary seals and pentacles on the appropriate day and burning incense made with the desired planetary influences in mind.

Mercury: The Liquid Carrier

Drawing techniques from spagyric alchemy, we are able to capture and maintain the energetic signature of the plant in liquid. This powerful preparation will contain the life force and consciousness of the plant.

The liquid vehicle is prepared by ritually harvesting fresh plant material on the day of the new moon before sunrise. This is when the subtle powers of the plant spirit are at their most potent. Approach the plant with offerings of incense, milk, honey, or wine, depositing them at the base of the plant.

Using a nonferrous implement, such as a copper blade or wooden wand, inscribe a circle around the plant counterclockwise to contain its virtue. Then harvest the aerial parts of the plant (flowers, stems, and leaves), traditionally using the left hand for occult purposes, in whatever amount works best for the size of the intended vessel. There isn't a specific amount that you'll need for your plant spirit vessel. Just collect whatever feels right.

Place the harvested plant material in your preconsecrated vessel. Cover it with vodka and allow it to macerate for an entire lunar cycle (essentially making a tincture). After this period, remove the plant material, pressing out all the liquid. Place the spent plant material in a clay vessel and burn it to ash. To further calcinate the ash and reduce it to an alchemical salt, spread it on a clay baking tray and place it in an oven set to high heat. Let it bake until it is a light gray-white color. Mix the ashes back into the alcohol (menstruum), and let the mixture macerate for another moon cycle. Then strain the mixture. You now have an energetically complete spagyric tincture containing the *tria prima*: salt, mercury, and sulphur, a liquid vessel of the plant's power.

Taking it a step further, you can add fresh leaves, flowers, seeds, stems, and roots so that all parts of the plant throughout all of its stages of life are present. These components can be added individually as they call to you, as an offering to the plant spirit vessel. You can do this over an entire season to create an elaborate bonding ritual with this plant spirit. The leaves and flowers are harvested in the summer, and the roots and seeds during the autumn.

If all you have is dried plant material or you aren't able to collect all the parts of a plant, you can still make a plant spirit vessel. If you need to skip the tincturing process or don't have extra plant material to make one, that is fine, too. As long as your vessel contains plant material and is ritually constructed in congress with your plant spirit familiar, it will be fine. As is the case for just about everything, the intention behind our actions is what matters. These suggestions are all additional layers of energy and power that enhance the vessel.

As long as the vessel remains sealed (when you're not adding or removing liquid) and out of direct sunlight, the tincture you've placed inside can last for years. You can, as you like, add a small amount of the spagyric liquid to fresh alcohol as a "starter" to repeat the process to create additional plant spirit vessels and carry on the same individual plant spirit's virtue.

Sulfur: Calling the Spirit into the Vessel

This ritual is just an example of how to call the power of the plant spirit into your vessel. You may feel called to enliven your vessel in a totally different way depending on your plant spirit and preferences. You should have already received your plant spirit's decision to reside here before constructing the vessel. Only a willing plant spirit is going to do this.

Arrange the vessel at the center of the altar, indoors or outdoors, during the dark moon. Leave the vessel open for the first part of the ritual. Surround it with candles and fresh plant material, or lay a triangle around it.

Get into a meditative state, and call out to the plant spirit in whatever way feels appropriate. Here's an example:

> *Back to the time when red and green were one,*
> *By the holy fire that feeds us both,*
> *I call out to my green brothers and sisters,*
> *By the dark fire that coils within.*
> *I call you up from below*
> *By the black sun and the hidden moon,*
> *Under the stars that made us both,*
> *I call you to this familiar place,*
> *So that red and green may again be one.*

Liquid Chlorophyll

Chlorophyll gives plants their green color and allows them to process sunlight into usable energy through photosynthesis. It is essentially the blood of the plant. Food-grade liquid chlorophyll is sold as a dietary supplement. It acts as an antioxidant and has a number of other potential benefits. It is dark emerald green and contains copper, which are the color and metal associated with Venus, planetary ruler of the natural world and herbal arts. I like to take chlorophyll as a supplement because it has a very high vibration and I can feel the green energy when I take it. It can also play a role in making and maintaining a plant spirit vessel. When calling a plant spirit into the vessel, add a few drops of liquid chlorophyll to the liquid inside as an offering. Once the spirit has entered the vessel, you can do on a regular basis. The chlorophyll will turn the liquid green if it isn't already, but it will settle to the bottom. You may or may not choose to add a drop of your own blood so that the two are mingled.

At this point you may choose to consume the herb in some way. This could be as a flower essence, anointing oil, ointment, incense, or smoking.

If you are going to smoke the herb, make sure it is safe to do so. (The nightshades are fine to smoke.) I would add 0.5 gram of the herb to a smoking blend and roll that up, but all you really need is a pinch. Inhale the smoke, and envision/feel the plant spirit slowly creep through you. Then, as you exhale, giving that breath back, blow the smoke toward the vessel. Do this three to five times, feeling the energy flow between you and the vessel.

Finishing Up

At this point the vessel is pretty much complete. You can continue with more ritual, do a plant spirit journey, or try scrying with the vessel. Keep the vessel on the altar or make a shrine for it. You can cover it with a cloth when it's not in use, like you would other spirit vessels. Bring out the plant spirit vessel whenever you want to connect with your plant spirit familiar. You can create multiple vessels for other familiar spirits as well. Don't forget to thank the plant spirit, maintain communication with it, and keep giving it offerings. If at some point you feel your work with that plant spirit is done, give the entire contents of the vessel back to the earth.

To incorporate the power of your plant spirit familiar, you can take a few drops of the liquid with water (depending on what plant you're using), or you can add it to other potions or incense blends to potentiate them.

Interact with the plant spirit vessel in the same way you would interact with the living plant. When you give offerings and communicate with it through visionary means, the vessel can serve as a touchstone to your plant spirit familiar.

Other Vessels

Alternatively, relics of bone or wood, including animal skulls, may serve as plant spirit familiar vessels. They can be vivified using inks, dyes, and tinctures made from the plant material. Keep such relics in a consecrated container, ideally a wooden box that is marked accordingly with sacred symbols. They may serve as oracular devices to assist with divination and spirit communication, removed from their resting place only when you are in direct communion with the plant spirit familiar.

Homunculi Smoke Incense

Use the smoke of this incense to activate and feed plant spirit vessels and glyphs as well as root fetishes. Blend the following herbs (in equal parts or as desired):

- Dandelion root
- Juniper berry
- Lemon balm
- Mandrake leaf
- Opoponax resin (or other sweet resin)
- Patchouli

CEREMONIAL BLENDS

These blends can be worked with by themselves or as part of a larger plant medicine ceremony. They can be called upon when extra assistance is needed to facilitate shifts. They can be infused into water and taken as tea, burned on charcoal as incense, or smoked in a pipe or papers. When rolled in papers, these blends can serve a dual function of calling upon plant allies and using the smoke as a smudge, using the smoke to direct your intention and move energy.

Cleansing and Purification

A tea and smoking blend for removing stagnant, low-vibration energy, spirits of disease, and unwanted influences. Blend equal parts of the following herbs:

- Lavender
- Mugwort
- Raspberry leaf
- Sage
- Skullcap
- Spearmint

Energy Shift and Support

A tea and smoking blend for uplifting energy, mood, and vibration for support during ceremony. Blend equal parts of the following herbs:

- Catnip
- Lemon balm
- Mullein
- Passionflower
- Tulsi
- Cannabis flower or CBD oil (optional)

Trickster's Secret Smoking Blend

Not for use as a tea; use as smoking blend or incense only. For opening the subtle senses to psychic working and spirit communication. This blend can also be used in ceremony to enhance the effects of other plant medicines. It can also be used for the Datura Entity Attachment Removal ritual (page 202).

- ✍ 0.5 gram *Amanita muscaria* cap (powdered)
- ✍ 0.5 gram blue lotus flower
- ✍ 0.5 gram *Datura stramonium*
- ✍ 0.5 gram skullcap

Spirit Smoke Offering: Stygian Incense

I resurrected this formula from the dead. It is specifically created for trafficking with the dead. It is inspired by ancient Greek myth and the boatman Charon. It contains herbs associated with and known to grow in graveyards, including dittany of Crete, mullein, and wild lettuce, among other necrobotanicals. It also contains the entheogenic seeds of black henbane, an herb historically connected to the realms of the dead, specifically the rivers said to flow there. This incense serves as a means of manifestation as well as bringing a visionary component. Use it to summon spirits of the dead or to journey to their realm. Burn small amounts to honor the dead and to aid in necromantic rituals.

Blend the following herbs (in equal parts or as desired):

- ✍ **Dittany of Crete**
- ✍ **Henbane leaf or seeds**
- ✍ **Mugwort**
- ✍ **Patchouli**
- ✍ **Skullcap**
- ✍ **Vervain**
- ✍ **Wild lettuce**

CHTHONIC ANOINTING OILS

Chthonic spirits are spirits of the Earth, terrestrial land spirits, the ancestral dead and familiar spirits. They also comprise the infernal or goetic spirits, the fallen angels, the entities connected to ancient and primal beliefs and deities. Each one has its own unique virtues or area of expertise that can be accessed in ritual using formulas made from herbs, resins, and oils that correspond to each spirit. These spirits have interesting connections to the plants of the poison path, and that is why I include formulas to connect with them here.

Invoke the energy of each spirit by chanting the spirit's associated names and focusing on the appropriate seal or sigil. Then burn the sigil, collect the ashes, and incorporate them into the base of each oil.

❀

Lilith Anointing Oil

Use this blend as a personal anointing oil or for ritual objects to evoke the spirit of Lilith, Malkah ha Shedim (Queen of Demons), and her legion of children. Lilith is connected to themes of personal sovereignty, sexual empowerment, domination, sending dreams/hag riding, breaking bonds, succubi, and psychic vampirism. She is a queer ally and enemy of the patriarchy and all it upholds.

Blend the following ingredients in a carrier oil of your choice, using just a few drops of the essential oils and tincture and a pinch of the hellebore and poppy seeds.

- Cassia essential oil
- Dragon's blood tincture
- Myrrh resin or essential oil
- Ylang-ylang essential oil
- A pinch of hellebore leaves
- A pinch of poppy seeds
- Ashes of symbols associated with Lilith
- Carrier oil of choice

Lucifer Anointing Oil

A mercurial blend created to connect with the Light-Bringer, rebellious teacher of humanity. Use it for summoning the spirits of air and for magic involving illumination, rebellion, groundbreaking workings, overcoming oppression, and occult power.

Blend the following ingredients in a carrier oil of your choice:

- Bay leaves and/or essential oil
- Fennel seeds and/or essential oil
- Lemongrass leaves and/or essential oil
- Mandrake leaves or tincture
- Ashes of Lucifer's sigil
- Carrier oil of choice

For this blend, I usually infuse the herbs (in dried form and equal parts) in the carrier oil and then add essential oils of the same plants when I divide the oil into smaller bottles.

Astaroth Anointing Oil

Use this anointing oil to summon Astaroth, patron spirit of occult pursuits, the daemonic force granting knowledge of past, present, and future. Astaroth aids in all intellectual pursuits, focusing the mind on one's intent. He can also be petitioned in rituals of love magic. Use this oil to anoint candles, seals, and the body and as a general anointing oil for connecting to this spirit.

Blend the following ingredients in a carrier oil of your choice:

- Camphor resin and/or essential oil
- Hibiscus flowers and/or essential oil
- Orris root powder
- Ashes of Astaroth's seal
- Carrier oil of choice

Stolas Anointing Oil

Stolas is quickly becoming a favorite familiar spirit of modern witches. Stolas, who often appears in the form of a raven, is known for teaching astronomy and the hidden virtues of stones and herbs, which makes them a perfect ally for the magical practitioner. Use this oil to anoint candles, seals, and the body and as a general anointing oil for connecting to this spirit.

Blend the following ingredients in a carrier oil of your choice:

- Cedarwood essential oil
- Centaury herb
- Sandalwood essential oil
- Solomon's seal root (just a few pieces in the bottle)
- Vervain herb or essential oil
- Crow, raven, or other black feather
- Ashes of Stolas's seal
- Carrier oil of choice

Azazel Anointing Oil

Azazel is a spirit associated with magic, rebellion, forbidden knowledge, and witchcraft. Azazel was a fallen angel, one of the Watchers mentioned in the Book of Enoch. Azazel and Shemyaza were associated with the fall of the Watcher angels, and Azazel was blamed for this and for disseminating forbidden knowledge. As a desert spirit, they are associated with the scapegoat of the Jewish Day of Atonement. Azazel, the scapegoat, was used as a vessel to contain all the sins of the people and was driven into the desert as a sacrifice (Leviticus 16). Azazel is specifically blamed with teaching humans how to build weapons of war. They are also linked to other "wicked" arts such as the use of cosmetics, jewelry making, and dye making (wearing colorful clothes was a sign of wickedness in the Old Testament). Azazel is also connected to the colorful "Peacock Angel" of the Yezidi people, a spirit of Luciferian gnosis. Azazel is a spirit of air and confers knowledge of all kinds. In witchcraft, Azazel is associated with Saturn/Capricorn/ the Horned God. Azazel's seal is the seal of the intelligence of Saturn, a planet intimately associated with witchcraft. A patron spirit of occult knowledge and Promethean rebellion, Azazel is a willing ally for occult pursuits. Azazel is a flamboyant and ostentatious spirit, representing the fabulousness that mainstream society scoffs at. Work with Azazel to connect with the Horned God and other patrons of the magical arts. Use this oil to anoint candles, seals, and the body and as a general anointing oil for connecting to this spirit.

Blend the following ingredients in a carrier oil of your choice:

- Blue tansy essential oil
- Cedarwood essential oil
- Mandrake leaf, root, or tincture
- Spikenard essential oil
- Vervain herb
- Vetiver essential oil
- Ashes of Azazel's seal
- Carrier oil of choice

HELPFUL WORKINGS FOR THE POISON PATH

Poison Bottle Warding Spell

From the Chinese five-poison formula to the putrid *scythicon* that struck fear in the hearts of ancient warriors, humankind has developed some truly terrible poisons. Battling by poison has an element of psychological warfare; for example, the Scythians made sure that everyone in the ancient world knew how terrible it was to die by their *scythicon*-poisoned arrows before a battle even began. In ancient times, there were specific rituals and rules regarding the containment and transport of poisonous substances. Many of these were physical safety measures with practical purposes, but others were more esoteric, based on the belief that these substances were malevolent in nature, capable of corrupting the air and killing from a distance. From such rituals arose the concept of a poison bottle.

Just like a traditional witch bottle contains nails, shards of glass, razors, and other sharp objects, the poison bottle is assembled using components with a baneful nature. You could combine this technique with a regular witch bottle construction, including sharp objects and your own urine for extra protective properties. The idea is to fill the bottle with components that are harmful, dangerous, deadly, and/or sharp and cover the bottle in protective, destructive, and baneful symbols. This creates a powerful apotropaic tool through sympathetic magic and the power of poison.

The bottle (or jar) can be whatever style you choose, but it should be something that seals completely because its contents are going to become pretty nasty.

On a night of the dark moon, begin filling the bottle with your ingredients, but no liquids—not yet. Wear gloves so you don't come into contact with anything you're adding, and cleanse yourself with incense or scented waters afterward.

Suggestions:

+ DEAD insects and spiders. Think: creepy crawly things with stingers, like centipedes, earwigs, ants, etc.
+ DEAD snakes, lizards, toads, and frogs.
+ Snake sheds, bones, or other animal remains.
+ Herbs with connections to death and dying: Spanish moss, mushrooms, devil's claw root, blackthorn pieces, herbs collected from a graveyard, etc.
+ Poisonous plants, meaning plants that are deadly, irritating, thorny or sharp, noxious, vining, or in some other way dangerous or difficult to control.
+ Toxic minerals (ones you wouldn't put in water), like malachite, selenite, etc.

Note: Do not kill any creatures to make a poison bottle. It is not necessary and won't help your working. Use only creatures that are found already dead. Alternatively, draw or paint images of these creatures on the outside of the jar or use plant material to represent the creatures whose energy you'd like to include.

Seal the bottle, then bury it in the earth until the next dark moon.

On the next dark moon, dig up the bottle. Add more ingredients if you like, and now fill the bottle with your own urine or vinegar. It sounds gross, and it is supposed to be.

Bury or hide the bottle near your front door or somewhere on your property. It will serve as protection from unwanted intrusions, act as an early warning system, and make sure that anything that does happen to cross the predetermined boundary will wish it hadn't.

In the presence of an enemy, poison bottles will slowly corrupt everything around them. Smaller jars can be made for this purpose, strengthened by the personal concerns of the target. Instead of filling the jar with urine, fill it with vinegar, castor oil, or mineral oil. The jar is then hidden in the proximity of the target. Some individuals would smash the jar on the target's doorstep for dramatic effect, but I don't condone that, of course.

❧ Henbane Ritual to Descend into Hel

This ritual was created for an underworld journey to the subterranean land of the dead, known in Norse mythology as Hel. This is not a place of evil or torture, like the Christian Hell. It is a realm of ancestral memory, primal creative forces, and the spirits of the land. Henbane has long been associated with the dead, specifically in communicating with them and in aiding their transition into the otherworld. We can work with this plant spirit as a guide on our own journey to retrieve ancestral knowledge or healing or to help a spirit with their transition into death.

This type of journey should not be undertaken lightly, and especially not for anyone in poor health. The idea is to return from the land of the dead when we are finished! Typically we'd take this type of journey only if a dire spiritual circumstance required intervention from the spirit world, and only in service of our community or to help someone in need. A spirit, for example, might need help transitioning, whether because they are afraid to move on or attached for some reason. By traveling ahead of them, we make it easier for them to do the same.

You will need:

> 4 large coins
> White sheet
> Incense burner and charcoal
> Henbane seeds, herb, or incense blend
> Funerary incense, such as myrrh resin
> Fragrant oils for anointing
> Ash (from charcoal, incense, etc.)

For this ritual, you will be preparing your body in a funerary manner to gain access to the ways of the psychopomp and death doula. First begin by lighting the charcoal disk in a fire safe dish or incense burner filled with sand. Myrrh resin, a traditional ingredient in embalming processes and funerary rites, can be burned throughout the ritual.

Set up all of the items on the floor in an area where you will be able to lie down. The first step is to wash your body, which could mean a shower or using a cloth and bowl of water to ritually wash yourself. Once you are clean, remain naked. Fumigate yourself with the smoke of myrrh resin and apply the fragrant oils of your choice. Dip your fingers in the ash and use it to draw a symbolic representation of a henbane flower (as best you can) on your chest.

Begin adding henbane to the charcoal, and carefully stand over the incense burner with the sheet around your shoulders (like a superhero cape). Say:

> *As the smoke rises, so shall my shade rise from my body*
> > *and meet the night.*
> *As I have marked myself, so shall the dead see me as*
> > *among their number.*
> *Baleful henbane, Devil's eye, I refuse my flesh, my spirit*
> > *flies.*

Allow the smoke to collect under the sheet briefly before wrapping the sheet around your legs and torso like a funerary shroud, keeping your arms free. Lie back on the floor. Keep the incense burner a safe distance away, but close enough that you can add more henbane and myrrh as you chant the words:

> *Hyoscyamus. Herba insana. Psychopompos chthonios. Spiritus meus descendit.*

Hold two of the coins in your left hand, or tuck them into the left side of your shroud. Do not lose them because you will need them to get back! The coins are a traditional payment for the various psychopomp spirits known for delivering the dead to their new homes. Place the other two coins on your eyelids. You will stay in this "resting" position, wrapped in the sheet and lying on the floor, while you complete your journey. Since you brought double payment and aren't actually dead, you can return from this journey anytime you want.

Continue chanting, with your arms down at your sides or crossed over your chest, until you feel you have achieved a sufficient state of relaxation. When you reach a point of silence, take a deep breath in, hold it for ten seconds, and then slowly exhale. Once you have exhaled all of your breath, wait as long as possible before inhaling again, and pay close attention to the silence and stillness. It is in this pocket of silence that you will find the door to the realm of the dead.

Become aware of your inner landscape. Where are you standing? Everyone perceives the land of the dead differently, and you may find yourself at the shore of a rushing river, in a warm field lit by a golden glow, or in a vast wasteland of shiny black stone. However, you perceive this landscape, know that this is the land of the dead. The visual journey you experience in this realm will be unique to you and to your reason for taking this journey in the first place. Spirits may approach you. You may have to complete a task or find something. Or you may encounter the spirits of your loved ones, both living and dead.

Once you feel you have achieved what you set out to do, bring your awareness to the two coins on your eyelids. Become aware of their heaviness, and as you do so, become aware of the weight of your physical body. Remove the coins from your eyelids and remove your shroud. Transfer one coin from your left hand to your right hand. Sit up, holding one coin in each hand as you settle back into your body.

⅍ *Belladonna Glamour Spell*

The nightshades are known for the hypnotic quality of their intoxication. They have been used in manipulative love magic and love potions since antiquity and are known for having aphrodisiac effects in small doses. In this ritual, you will tap into the very real power that belladonna has to bewitch, entrance, and dominate. The purpose is to create an aura of irresistibility to attract and influence. You can also use it to go under the radar and get into situations you normally wouldn't be able to by blending in and making people feel comfortable.

   You will need:

> 5 purple chime candles
> I black chime candle
> **Belladonna-infused anointing oil or ointment**
> **Belladonna plant material**
> **Black onyx stone or sphere or obsidian mirror**

   Anoint the candles with the belladonna oil or ointment, applying it from wick to base. Arrange the purple candles in a pentagram pattern. You might set them up on the altar as a focal point or on the floor in a spot large enough for you to sit or lie down. Place some of the plant material at the base of each candle, and in the center place the onyx in whatever form you have it. Now light all the candles, including the black one. Holding the black candle, walk the perimeter of the circle or trace a circle in the air above the altar with your arms while chanting:

> *Sovereign lady of the night, hear my beckon call,*
> *Catch their eyes, bend the light, my every move enthrall.*
> *By dark of night and blackest moon, wrapped in ebon cloak,*
> *Sharpened blade and spinning loom, desire I evoke.*
> *Hear me ancient plant of fate, your power please bestow.*
> *I call the lady of death's gate, within the circle show.*

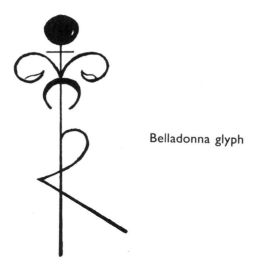

Belladonna glyph

Place the black candle inside the circle of purple candles, and anoint your temples, third eye, heart, and wrists with belladonna oil. You could also trace the belladonna glyph onto your body using the oil, ointment, ash, or other pigment. If the circle is large enough, carefully enter it and pick up the black stone/sphere/mirror. Imagine a violet-black flame emanating from the candles into the stone and into you. Chant the following words until you reach a trance state or until the candles burn down:

Atropos kthonios, herba lamiarum, herba diaboli invoco en
noctum est.

Afterward, keep the black stone/sphere/mirror in a safe place, away from sunlight and wrapped in cloth or kept in a pouch or box. Only take the object out at night during the dark moon to recharge the spell by repeating both chants and holding the object. Anoint your palms with belladonna oil or dust them with belladonna plant material before removing the object from its container. In the same way, anoint your palms and temples before interacting with those you wish to influence with your femme fatale aura.

ॐ Belladonna Heart of a Harpy Spell

A spell for ferocity and empowerment when you are going into difficult situations or coming up against opposition.

One of the common names for *Atropa belladonna* in Germanic languages is Valkyrie berry (*walkerbeere*) or Valkyrie tree (*walkerbaum*). In Norse mythology, the Valkyries are powerful and fierce female spirits; after a battle, they bring half of the slain warriors to their hall to await Ragnarok. The Valkyries are in alignment with belladonna's martial aspects. The plant is associated with the Roman war goddess Bellona, and the berries were once used by hunters to increase their perception and hunting ability. As late as the nineteenth century, German hunters would still often consume three or four belladonna berries before going out hunting (Rätsch 2005, 82), a practice that was said to help them hunt like the wolf, an apex predator. In fact, belladonna was also known as wolf cherry and many other names associating it with Odin's animal spirit. Belladonna brings an unmatched ferocity, activates our instincts, and pushes us to survive no matter what the cost.

In this ritual, you will tap into the warrior spirit of the Valkyries for confronting enemies, overcoming obstacles, and standing in your power against the adversarial forces of oppression. Perform this ritual to gain clear sight in the darkness, to uncover what needs to be seen or what is lurking in the darkness. This ritual can help you connect with your ancestors for strength, resolve, and divine protection from warrior spirits.

You will need:

> **Drum or other percussive instrument (this could be a staff you tap on the ground or two sticks you tap together)**
> **Belladonna in a form that can be used for pigment (fresh berries and/or belladonna infusion, oil, or ointment mixed with activated charcoal)**

This is a very simple ritual, and it could be enhanced by performing an entheogenic sacrament beforehand, consuming entheogenic plant material or using entheogenic incense, a flying ointment, or other means of entering trance. For example, I would apply belladonna flying ointment to the soles of my feet, my chest, and the back of my neck to begin the ritual, using meditative techniques or breathwork to connect with this plant ally. Once you have entered a sufficient trance state through your preferred means, you will mark yourself for battle, marking yourself as other so that you can stand with the spirits.

Prepare your pigment: smash the berries to release their dark juices, or mix a belladonna extraction with activated charcoal to darken it.

Take your drum or other instrument and beat or tap it, producing an increasingly fast and loud rhythm to raise the energy and call the warrior spirits in your line. Your intention is to raise your adrenaline level and make your heart speed faster, so think marching into battle!

Once you feel the energy is appropriate, use your belladonna pigment to draw the six-spoked wheel or *hagalaz* rune at the center of your check or over your heart. It looks like an X with a vertical line through it (see figure, page 137), and it is one of the most important and powerful runes, associated with the destructive force of hail and the inevitable power of the Nornir.

As you trace the three lines of this rune with your fingers, visualize its shape in your mind's eye and intone the name of the rune, drawing out the vowels with deep breaths: "Haaaaagaaaaalaaaazzz." Beat your drum again while you do this, and allow yourself to fall into a rhythm for a few moments. Visualize an open field, an ancient battleground. All of the dead are long since gone and buried, but you hear the sounds of the battle like it is happening right now. Hear the clash of swords and shields. Hear the crash of lightning and thunder over the battlefield, which opens the sky to a cloud of wings belonging to a group of warrior women: the Valkyries.

Hold this image in your mind's eye and continue to hear the drum beating with the rhythm of your heart. Now you can begin painting yourself with other markings. This can be left to your intuition; perhaps you will be led to draw lines under your eyes or mouth, or perhaps something more abstract will emerge.

When you have finished marking yourself, pick up your drum and continue beating it, allowing it to raise the energy around you. As you feel the ritual begin to come to a close, you can naturally begin to slow the beat of the drum and return to a more relaxed state of consciousness.

When you have finished with the ritual, leave some belladonna berries, mead, wine, or other offerings out for the Valkyries and the spirit of belladonna.

Valkyrie Names/Titles

Here is a short list of the specific Valkyries I like to work with. Many of these names are found in the Poetic Edda.

Brinhildr: a leader of the Valkyrie; her name means "bright armor"

Eir: associated with medicine, healing, and herbalism

Göndu: wand wielder

Herfjötur: a powerful Valkyrie known for her ability to place "war fetters"

Hervör alvitr: an all-wise, strange creature

Skuld: a Valkyrie and also a Norn; is associated with the future, her name meaning "debt" or "obligation"

❧ Datura Entity Attachment Removal

Datura is a powerful ally for the removal of parasitic entities, harmful energy attachments, and unwelcome spirits. When incorporated into rituals of cleansing and purification, datura brings a powerful ability to transmute spiritual "toxins" and heal the unseen sources of disharmony.

For this ritual you will need a living datura plant that is in bloom, but if you don't have one, you can find other ways to incorporate the spirit of datura. You can perform this ritual for yourself or for another person.

You will need:

I living datura plant

A small amount of dried datura leaves

Incense burner and charcoal

Copal or other lunar incense/herbs for offering

A bowl of rain/spring/moon water

Ideally, the entire ritual will be performed outdoors. This is partly due to needing a well-ventilated area for the datura we will be burning. However, it can be completed indoors once the flowers have been collected.

Approach the datura plant at nighttime when it is in bloom. Light the charcoal and burn the copal or other offertory incense for the datura spirit and tell it why you are there. Ask the plant spirit for its help in removing this entity, saying:

> Grandmother, once you were a warrior.
> You fought battles too old to remember their names.
> Now you are a healer, a medicine woman.
> Tonight I come in darkness followed by another.
> I ask you to take up your spear once more, and sing your healing
>   songs for [person's name].
> Grandmother who can heal and harm, fight by my side tonight
>   to defeat this foe.

Collect three open datura flowers, offering prayers of thanks and more incense. (Once you have collected the flowers, you can remain outside with the datura plant or finish the ritual indoors if necessary.)

Add a small pinch of dried datura leaves to the charcoal, allowing it to burn, filling the space with the spirit of datura.

Holding the three datura flowers together, dip their open ends in the bowl of water. Use them to sweep the body with a brushing motion, on the front and the back, beginning at the top of the head, moving to the shoulders and arms, and working your way down the torso and down each leg, sweeping the energy outward as if you were dusting something off. While you do this, ask the datura spirit to remove and transmute all impurities, imbalances, and disruptive forces.

When you are done sweeping the body, place the datura flowers in the bowl of water and thank the datura spirit for its help and healing.

Add more dried datura leaves to the charcoal. Carefully use it to trace the entire body of the person, allowing smoke to reach all the extremities. Take care so the person does not inhale large amounts of smoke. While you do this, ask the datura spirit to remove any blockages and to lift any harmful spiritual influences with the smoke.

When you are done, dip your hands in the bowl of water. Place your wet hands on either side of the person's head and gently slide your hands downward, wiping the water on the person. Repeat this process with each arm and leg. (If you are doing this on yourself, use one hand to do the opposite arm and leg and vice versa.) Finally, with your fingers, lightly sprinkle the water on their torso and also on the ground around them. While you do this, ask the datura spirit to help wash away any contamination and malevolent forces with the water.

If it feels necessary, you can repeat any step of the process, and you can repeat the entire ritual for situations that require persistence. If you are unable to perform one of the steps, you can still perform parts of the ritual effectively. When you have completed the cleansing with flowers, smoke, and water, return the flowers and any remaining water to the base of the living datura plant, giving thanks for its partnership and support.

❧ Amulet of Night Eternal (for Solar Protection)

I have had a sensitivity to the direct sunlight since I can remember, and I wrote this ritual about ten years ago to create an amulet of protection against photosensitivity and the fatigue, nausea, and dizziness that come with it. I include the ritual in this book because I have found that working with baneful spirits can sometimes leave a person feeling drained or sensitive to light, which is interesting when we consider the chemical action of tropane alkaloids and eyesight. Tropane alkaloids have a mydriatic effect, which means that they dilate the pupils allowing more light to come in. This also works on an esoteric level opening our spiritual sight to be more perceptive. This amulet will provide some extra protection and balance when we are traveling between dark and light.

For this ritual, I turned to the powers of the elements, watchtowers, and spirits of the night, including that of datura, a night-blooming flower. The ritual calls for a dried datura flower, but you could also use a datura ointment or oil to anoint the amulet, the candles, and your body. The amulet can be any piece of jewelry or object that you can carry with you. I also still have the silver and labradorite pendant that I used the first time I cast this spell, and I am wearing it now.

You will need:

A piece of jewelry or wearable charm as the amulet

Black or dark-colored stones (enough to create an outline
   around the altar)

4 violet candles

2 large black candles

1 large white candle

Offertory incense (equal parts jasmine flowers, mugwort, and
   wormwood ground to a fine consistency)

1 dried datura flower, collected at night preferably during the
   dark moon

Set the two black candles on either side of the white candle on the altar.
Light the white candle. Light the incense, and keep it replenished on the altar or
eastern point of the circle. Place the dark stones at the quarters, or use them
to create a circle boundary or a smaller circle on top of the altar if you have
fewer stones.

While the incense burns, engrave each of the four violet candles with the
runes *algiz* ᛉ and *isa* ᛁ. Then light the candles and place them at the quarters
of the circle or on top of the altar if you are working with a smaller area. Place
the amulet in the center of the altar, or put it on if it can be worn.

Now, face north or go to the northern point of the circle and say:

> I call upon the wind of the north, land of greatest darkness,
> Cold wind, wind of death.
> Lend me your power.
> Energy of the deep dark Earth, shadows from below,
> Lend me power from your dark depths.
> Uriel of the dark night,
> Cast your shadow upon this vessel.

Turn to face east or go to the eastern point of the circle and say:

> I call upon you, element of air,
> Wind of the east,
> Bringer of storms that blot out the sun.
> Guide the darkness to me tonight,

Raziel, keeper of secrets,
Whisper your incantations over this vessel.
And the many-colored rays of Azazel,
Be the light that shines brightest.

At the south:

Cassiel, come to me and join our circle of night.
May your dark wings fan the flames.
Wind of the south, come with warm embrace.
Saturnian spirit, keeper of night's gate,
Dark flame that burns within all,
Consecrate this vessel with your darkness.
Elemental fire, I conjure thee.

To the west:

Gabriel, in the west, whose winds we call,
Come to my circle from the
Land of the setting sun.
Rise on black waves,
Deep and dark as the sky.
Bless this vessel with your waters.

Return and stand facing the altar. Light the two black candles and say:

Elements four, elements prime,
Gather at this occulted time,
Transformed beneath the dark sky,
Different creatures without the sun's eye.
Dark watchers of the night, descend.
With your power, shadow's protection lend.
By this token that I bear,
Water, fire, earth, and air,
Turn the sun's spears away.
By Isa and Algiz,

I freeze its burning rays.
I call upon the queen of the night,
The spirit of datura, moon's flower,
Hekate, and the countless goddesses
Of nocturnal luminaries.
With this amulet
May I feel the cool kiss of night,
Even during the brightest of days.
May I always find the shade,
Even when the sun is high.

Return to the purple candle in the north. Blow or snuff out the candle while saying:

Spirits of the north,
In darkness you came,
In darkness you part.
Thank you for your
Help in my nocturnal art.

Repeat this at the east, south, and west, putting out all the purple candles, and then return to face the altar. Blow or snuff out the white candle in the center, leaving the two black candles to burn. Remove the amulet from your neck if you are wearing it and place it upon the altar, saying:

All began in darkness, and to the darkness all shall return.

Let the amulet sit there as the black candles burn so it can soak up the night, but put the amulet back on before the sun comes up on the first day. The amulet can be recharged by taking the stones that you used to create the circle and putting them in a box with the amulet, or put them in a bowl and cover with a dark cloth. Put the box/bowl out under the night sky for three nights in a row, bringing it inside before sunrise and keeping it out of the daylight during those three days. After that the amulet can be taken back out and worn, doing this however often you feel is necessary.

❀

Datura and Tobacco Initiatory Salve

Recently I was asked to create a strong formula for an initiatory ritual in which only a small amount of ointment would be used to draw a symbol on the participant. So I made something stronger than normal. Datura and tobacco are powerful plant allies and often used together. Datura is often viewed as a grandmother spirit and tobacco as a grandfather. Both plants have infinite ancestral wisdom to teach us, and when we work with them together they have a very special synergy.

You will need:

- 8 grams dried *Datura stramonium* seeds
- 1 tablespoon alcohol (I used datura tincture for extra strength)
- 60 ml datura-infused oil (in a 1:10 ratio)
- 2 grams dried *Nicotiana rustica*, powdered
- 10 grams carnauba wax
- A pinch of ash

Grind the dried datura seeds, being careful *not* to breathe the dust. (I recommend using a coffee grinder that is reserved for powerful plants like this. You don't want datura in your coffee!)

Transfer the ground-up seeds to a small glass container and add enough alcohol to cover them. (I used an existing tincture made with fresh datura. The tincture ratio wasn't terribly important because I used it mainly for its alcohol content and extra alkaloids.) Let the seeds sit until they absorb the alcohol. Stir.

Stir the alcohol-soaked seeds into the datura-infused oil. Warm in a double boiler (it gets hot very fast with a small amount of oil like this, so go slow with the temperature). When the alcohol starts bubbling to the surface of the oil, reduce the heat and stir for just a few minutes. All of the alkaloids are already extracted, so you're just getting things hot and thoroughly mixed. Then remove from the heat.

Let the oil cool slightly, and then add the powdered tobacco, stirring it in. Let the mixture sit until it is cool. Wearing gloves, strain the oil. You should end up with about 50 ml.

Set a glass container on a scale and tare its weight. Pour in the oil and note its weight; you should have around 40 grams. Add one-quarter part wax (about 10 grams). Add a pinch of powdered hardwood ash (horticultural ash, or you can make your own). Heat in a double boiler until the wax is melted. Mix well, pour into a container for storage, and let cool.

❧ *Syrian Rue Hex-Breaker*

This spell can be performed to break any spells or unwanted influences on the person who casts it. It can be employed to avert the evil eye, all forms of maleficia, and any spiritual and energetic attachments. Syrian rue has long been known for its spiritual powers. In Pakistan it is burned to break the enchantments of djinn and avert evil spirits, and in Turkey it is used as an incense to remove the evil eye (Rätsch 2005).

You will need:

4 white candles
1–2 grams *Peganum harmala* seeds
Incense burner and charcoal
A shot glass of saltwater

Light the charcoal for the incense burner. Light the four candles and arrange them in a cross with yourself in the center. Add a small amount of Syrian rue seeds to the charcoal, holding the shot glass of saltwater over the smoke. Then take the shot glass to each of the four candles and say:

> *Cleansed by the waters and purified in fire. All corruption*
> *and ill intent is banished from me.*

Now, standing at the center of the four candles, take a small pinch of Syrian rue seeds, place them on your tongue, and say, "Besasa." *Besasa* means plant of Bes, an ancient Egyptian apotropaic deity associated with Syrian rue. Make sure you say the name while the seeds are in your mouth. Then take a tiny sip of water from the shot glass and quickly turn your head to the left and spit out the water and the seeds. Repeat this, spitting out seeds and water to your right, behind you, and in front of you.

For added potency, you might put something to represent the hex being broken on the ground in front of you, such as an egg, peanut, or small breakable bottle (make sure you wear shoes and do this outside). As you make the last motion of spitting in front of yourself, step forward at the same time and crush the object on the ground. The physical action of breaking the object along with the sound and sensation will help reinforce the intention of the spell.

Let the candles burn down and leave an offering to the deity Bes. According to the late Christian Rätsch, Bes was a dwarf spirit that was beloved by the ancient Egyptians as a protector. Rätsch says that small statues and images of the god were fumigated with Syrian rue seeds to activate their protective powers (Rätsch 2005, 426).

ও Yew Tree Self-Sacrifice

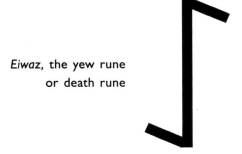

Eiwaz, the yew rune
or death rune

Yew is the death tree. It is represented by the death rune, *eiwaz*, and is one of the trees identified as the world tree. All parts of the yew are toxic except for its berry-like arils; its alkaloids are even used in cancer treatments. The yew is connected to the myth of the sacrificed god or shamanic death. For support during periods of extreme change and upheaval, or when transformative changes are needed, we can approach the spirit of yew to help with the process of shedding and mourning parts of ourselves and our lives that no longer serve us.

In this exercise, we will call upon the spirit of the yew tree and sacrifice parts of ourselves to our self, as the gods have done before us. We shed these parts of ourselves for knowledge, power, perspective, healing, and growth. This is a very individual process for everyone, but we all have things worth sacrificing.

Find a yew tree. It doesn't have to be in a graveyard, but it can be. Sit beneath it, preferably with your back against its trunk. Contemplate the parts of yourself that you would be willing to sacrifice. What would you happily be rid of?

Then ask yourself, is there any part of you that would be too great a sacrifice? What parts of yourself or your identity are you so attached to that you would deny yourself the opportunity to grow into something more? What do these parts mean to you? Why does letting go of them seem like it would mean your demise?

Finding where these fears lie and what is at the root of them helps you understand your inner motivations better and makes it easier to let go of things when you no longer need them. Just because you let go of something or someone doesn't mean that it can't come back to you, and allowing yourself to be free opens you to so much more potential.

The greatest transformations do not come without a price, and when you come to the spirits and offer what you hold dear, they take your prayers more seriously. Maybe there is something you want to bring into your life, and you need to make room for it. Maybe there is something you are desperately trying to be rid of, but you are unwilling to begin letting go to shift things in a new direction. Call these things to mind and hold them up before yourself. Feel the firmness of the yew tree against you. Touching its wood awakens the spirit within. Ask that it help you in shedding this part of yourself, giving it to the tree as an offering. You may also choose to make an offering of smoke, a libation, or a drop of your blood on the tree.

This can be a place you return to in order to strengthen your bond with the spirit of yew. From its fertile soil, fed by the corpses of all you have left behind, you can grow the garden of your wildest dreams.

Remember, sacrifice is a serious thing, even if it is a symbolic sacrifice to yourself. We don't always see the full scope of what we are giving up, but we must trust that on the other side is something greater than what we let go.

The following is a petition you can say when sitting in meditation with the yew tree:

> *Sentry of death, door of rebirth,*
> *Forming within your inner chamber,*
> *I lay here all that has passed from me,*
> *Feeding the dead with your roots.*
> *Rex nemorensis, sacrificed gods,*
> *I leave with you [name/situation/quality you are*
> *   leaving behind]*
> *So that I may grow eternally*
> *From the inside out, just as yew.*

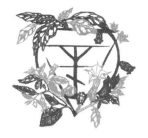

Final Words

(hopefully not my last)

*T*he poison path can be many different things, depending on who you ask, and its ideas can be incorporated into your spiritual practice in just as many ways. The place where I found myself on this path is not the same place where I find myself now, and as with any living thing, it grows and changes with time and attention. One thing is sure: This highly individualistic approach to plant spirit practices, natural medicine, and green witchery strikes a chord within all of us, in one way or another. By drawing us in for a closer look, or bringing up to the surface that which we fear, it gives us an opportunity to take a closer look at ourselves and the world around us. The plants (and fungi) of this path are mirrors, and what we see reflected back to us is not always what we would expect, nor is it always what we would wish to see. We can take many different approaches to explore the wisdom and power these allies have to offer, whether it is for clinical purposes or spiritual pursuits, or, as many come to realize, a combination of the two.

This is my understanding and my personal gnosis. It is where this winding and often obscured path has led me thus far, and I have only just begun to understand what these beautiful and terrific spirits have to teach those who are willing to take that first step. I am one voice among many who are collectively singing the songs of these not-so-forgotten plant spirits. Not everyone will choose to delve this far into occult herbalism or poison plant medicine, and that is okay too. I hope that you found something of value within these pages, something that has inspired you to think differently about how you work with plants in your own practice. It is my goal to present to you, the reader, the idea that the word *poison* can mean many different things, just like the word *witch*. From my perspective, *poison* is a signpost to tell us that there is more to be discovered if we choose to take a closer look, and that if we can resist the urge to turn away immediately in fear or disgust, we will be shown a clearer picture of the world we live in and our own place in it.

As we've discussed throughout this book, the plants of the poison path are often called baneful, which generally means harmful. Harmful to what, you might wonder? To the status quo? To a rigidly fixed understanding of what plants we should work with and how? To a society that labels and categorizes all things in an attempt to control the wild parts of the world? To a society that has forgotten that they are still a part of nature? If the poison path has taught me one thing, it is that things are never what they seem, and there is always something lurking beneath the surface, waiting to be discovered. Like Eve, who dared to take that first bite of the fruit of knowledge, we must always continue to question and to learn more.

As always, banefully yours,
Coby Michael

Works Cited

Allaun, Chris. 2022. *Underworld: Shamanism Myth and Magic*. Mandrake of Oxford.

Belanger, Michelle. 2004. *The Psychic Vampire Codex: A Manual of Magick and Energy Work*. Weiser Books.

Björn, Albert. 2023. *Icelandic Plant Magic: Folk Herbalism of the North*. Crossed Crow Books.

Boyer, Corinne. 2017. *Plants of the Devil*. Three Hands Press.

Boyer, Corinne. 2021. *The Witch's Cabinet: Plant Lore, Sorcery and Folk Magic*. Three Hands Press.

Dominguez Jr., Ivo. 2022. *Presentation on: Dark and Primal Deities and Spirits*. Shared with permission.

Emboden, William A. 1974. *Bizarre Plants: Magical, Monstrous, Mythical*. MacMillan Publishing Co.

Folkard, Richard. 1884. *Plant Lore, Legends and Lyrics: Embracing the Myths, Traditions, Superstitions and Folklore of the Plant Kingdom*. Folkard and Son.

Frater Tenebris. 2022. *The Philosophy of Dark Paganism: Wisdom & Magick to Cultivate the Self*. Llewellyn Worldwide.

Fries, Jan. 1993. *Helrunar: A Manual of Rune Magick*. Mandrake of Oxford.

Frisvold, Nikolaj de Mattos. 2014. *Craft of the Untamed: An Inspired Vision of Traditional Witchcraft*. Mandrake of Oxford.

Frisvold, Nikolaj de Mattos. 2021. *Trollrún: A Discourse of Trolldom and Runes in the Northern Tradition*. Hadean Press.

Gary, Gemma. 2021. *The Devil's Dozen: Thirteen Craft Rites of the Old One*. Troy Books.

Gellis, Roberta. 2003. *Lucrezia Borgia and the Mother of Poisons*. Forge Books.

Gibbs, Frederick. 2019. *Poison, Medicine, and Disease in Late Medieval and Early Modern Europe*. Routledge.

Ginzburg, Carlo. 2004. *Ecstasies: Deciphering the Witches' Sabbath.* University of Chicago Press.

Grieve, Maud. 1931. *A Modern Herbal.* New York: Dover Publications.

Hansen, Harold. 1983. The Witch's Garden (Translated from Danish by Muriel Crofts originally titled *Heksens Urtegard*). Samuel Weiser, Inc.

Hatsis, Thomas. 2015. *The Witches' Ointment: The Secret History of Psychedelic Magic.* Park Street Press.

Hatsis, Thomas. 2018. *Psychedelic Mystery Traditions: Spirit Plants, Magical Practices, Ecstatic States.* Park Street Press.

Herman, Eleanor. 2019. *The Royal Art of Poison: Fatal Cosmetics, Deadly Medicines and Murder Most Foul.* Duckworth UK.

Hohman, John George. 2010 (orig. pub. 1828). *Pow-Wows or Long Lost Friend: A Collection of Mysterious and Invaluable Arts and Remedies, for Man as Well as Animals.* Wildside Press.

Hubbard, Ben. 2019. *Poison: The History of Potions, Powders and Murderous Practitioners.* Carlton Publishing Group.

Inkwright, Fez. 2021. *Botanical Curses and Poisons: The Shadow Lives of Plants.* Liminal 11.

Jackson, Nigel Aldcroft. 1994. *Call of the Horned Piper.* Capal Bann Publishing.

Jarving, Stein. 2004. "Sámi Shamanism." *Eutopia Adventure*, June 16, 2004.

Konstantinos. 2005. *Nocturnicon: Calling Dark Forces and Powers.* Llewellyn Worldwide.

Lecouteaux, Claude. 2010. *The Secret History of Vampires: Their Multiple Forms and Hidden Purposes.* Inner Traditions.

Lindequist, Ulrike. 1992. Datura. In *Hagers Handbuch der pharmazeutischen Praxis*, 5th ed., 4:1138–54. Berlin: Springer.

Liu, Yan. 2021. *Healing with Poisons: Potent Medicines in Medieval China.* University of Washington Press.

Masha, M.D. Baba. 2002. *Microdosing with Amanita Muscaria: Creativity, Healing, and Recovery with the Sacred Mushroom.* Park Street Press.

Mayor, Adrienne. 2003. *Greek Fire, Poison Arrows, and Scorpion Bombs: Biological and Chemical Warfare in the Ancient World.* Overlook Duckworth.

McNeill, William H. 1976. *Plagues and Peoples.* Anchor Books.

Michael, Coby. 2021. *The Poison Path Herbal.* Inner Traditions.

Monmouth, John of. 2012. *Genuine Witchcraft Is Explained: The Secret History of the Royal Windsor Coven and the Regency.* Capall Bann Publishing.

Oates, Shani. 2022. *The Hanged God: Ódin Grímnir.* Anathema Publishing.

Pearson, Nicholas. 2022. *Flower Essences from the Witch's Garden: Plant Spirits in Magical Herbalism.* Destiny Books.

Rankin, Alisha. 2021. *The Poison Trials: Wonder Drugs, Experiment and the Battle for Authority in Renaissance Science.* University of Chicago Press.

Rätsch, Christian. 2005. *The Encyclopedia of Psychoactive Plants: Ethnopharmacology and Its Applications.* Park Street Press.

Rätsch, Christian, and Claudia Müller-Ebeling. 2005. *The Encyclopedia of Aphrodisiacs: Psychoactive Substances for Use in Sexual Practices.* Park Street Press.

Rogers, Robert Dale. 2014. *The Devil May Care: Herbs of the Underworld.* Prairie Deva Press.

Schulke, Daniel. 2018. *Veneficium: Magic, Witchcraft and the Poison Path.* 2nd rev. ed. Three Hands Press.

Sédir, Paul. 2021. *Occult Botany: Sédir's Concise Guide to Magical Plants.* Trans. R. Bailey. Inner Traditions.

Sidky, Homayun. 1997. *Witchcraft, Lycanthropy, Drugs, and Disease: An Anthropological Study of the European Witch-Hunt.* Peter Lang Group.

Somerset, Anne. 2014. *The Affair of the Poisons: Murder, Infanticide and Satanism in the Court of Louis XIV.* St. Martin's Press.

Stevens, Serita Deborah, and Anne Klarner. 1990. *Deadly Doses: A Writer's Guide to Poisons.* Writer's Digest.

Thompson, C. J. S. 1924 (orig. pub. 1899). *Poison Mysteries in History, Romance and Crime.* J. B. Lippincott Company.

Watts, D. C. 2007. *Elsevier's Dictionary of Plant Lore.* Elsevier Inc.

Westbrooks, Randy G., and James W. Preacher. 1986. *Poisonous Plants of Eastern North America.* University of South Carolina.

Williams, Joshua. 2022. *The Green Arte: The Craft of the Herbwise.* Aeon Books.

Index